The Oblique View

Cardiology from a different angle

Michael S Norell MD FRCP

tfm Publishing Limited, Castle Hill Barns, Harley, Nr Shrewsbury, SY5 6LX, UK, Tel: +44 (0)1952 510061; Fax: +44 (0)1952 510192
E-mail: nikki@tfmpublishing.com; Web site: www.tfmpublishing.com

Design & Typesetting: Nikki Bramhill
Front cover image & cartoons: © 2007 Steve Yentis

First Edition © 2007
ISBN: 978 1 903378 53 3

Acknowledgement
The material within this book has been reproduced with kind permission from the publishers of:

1. *Cardiology News* © 2005-2007 Pinpoint Scotland Ltd. (www.pinpointmedical.com).
2. *British Journal of Cardiology* © 2004-2007 Medinews (Cardiology) Ltd. (www.bjcardio.com).

Printed by Gutenberg Press Ltd., Gudja Road, Tarxien, PLA 19, Malta. Tel: +356 21897037; Fax: +356 21800069.

Contents

Acknowledgements

The British Cardiovascular Intervention Society (BCIS) put the first of these articles (on music in the cardiac catheter laboratory) into its newsletter. This publication was discontinued shortly afterwards (no connection) when their website took over.

Henry Purcell was then kind enough to use subsequent articles in a regular column (The Oblique View) in the *British Journal of Cardiology*. I acknowledge his support and encouragement together with that of Kate White, Jackie Cooper and all the editing and production team at MediNews (Cardiology).

Clive Weston was also sufficiently farsighted to publish other essays of mine as a regular feature (Added Sounds) in *Cardiology News*, before he stood down as Editor (no connection there, either). I much appreciate his help and that of Jenny Fallon and all her colleagues at Pinpoint Scotland.

The ideas for many of these chapters were developed whilst walking my dog, a Weimaraner, called Nelson; I felt therefore that he should also get a mention.

I am sincerely grateful for the interest, enthusiasm and support of my publisher, Nikki Bramhill, and for the contribution that Steve Yentis has made with his unique cartoons. I particularly wish to express thanks to my secretary, Helen Godfrey, for her constant, unfailing and enthusiastic support. How she has put up with me for the last few years I shall never know.

Finally, I thank the occasional readers who have contacted me from time to time just to let me know that some of my observations resonate with their own views. It is reassuring that I am not alone and that my efforts have been read at least by someone other than me.

Dr. Michael S. Norell MD FRCP
Consultant Interventional Cardiologist,
The Heart and Lung Centre,
Wolverhampton.

May 2007

Author biography

Michael Norell was born and brought up in North London and qualified in medicine at University College Hospital. Having trained in cardiology he left the capital for a consultant post in Hull and subsequently moved to the West Midlands in order to set up the new angioplasty service in the Heart and Lung Centre at Wolverhampton. His twenty-five year involvement in percutaneous coronary intervention has provided more than a few insights into the workings of the cardiological mind.

He still maintains a passing interest in the fortunes of Tottenham Hotspur but his football allegiance has moved largely to Wolverhampton Wanderers. A favourite pastime is sailing but as he lives in a small village on the Shropshire/Staffordshire border his yacht, "Heart Sound" - moored on the River Orwell, near Ipswich - is sadly underused.

Abbreviations

ACS Acute coronary syndrome

ACT Activated clotting time

AMI Acute myocardial infarction

AR Aortic regurgitation

AV Atrioventricular

CABG Coronary artery bypass grafting

CCU Coronary care unit

CHD Coronary heart disease

CHF Chronic heart failure

DCA Directional coronary atherectomy

EDP End-diastolic pressure

EEG Electroencephalogram

ESM Ejection systolic murmur

IHT Inter-hospital transfer

JVP Jugular venous pressure

LAD Left anterior descending

LAO Left anterior oblique

LVH Left ventricular hypertrophy

MR Mitral regurgitation

MVR Mitral valve repair

NAD Nothing abnormal detected

NICE National Institute for Health and Clinical Excellence

NSF National service framework

PCI Percutaneous coronary intervention

PCT Primary Care Trust

PERLA Pupils equal and reactive to light

PTCA Percutaneous transluminal coronary angioplasty

TCT Transcatheter cardiovascular therapeutics

TR Tricuspid regurgitation

VF Ventricular fibrillation

VPB Ventricular premature beats

VSD Ventricular septal defect

Dedication

To Niki,

Ellie, Matthew and Charlie

Chapter 1

I'll never forget 'what's his name'

It was Richard Asher (medical author and father of one of Paul McCartney's early girlfriends) who noted that clinical conditions tend to become recognised only when they are named. Indeed, his own application of 'Munchausen' to the unfortunates who generate symptoms in order to obtain medical care, is a notable example. We all struggled with these at medical school, trying to differentiate Murphy's, from McBurney's, sign and ensuring that the Paterson-(Brown)-Kelly-Plummer-Vinson syndrome was expressed in the right order.

Browsing through a collection of such eponyms is enlightening, not least because one finds that even commonplace phenomena appear to have acquired someone's surname. Thus, Pins sign (after E. Pins, Austrian physician, 1845-1913) describes the loss of pericardial pain when leaning forwards. One also discovers signs of which one was totally unaware: the ease with which heart sounds can be heard over the abdomen, following rupture of an abdominal viscus, was described by Claybrook (initials E.B., US surgeon, 1871-1931; I bet you knew that).

During my surgical house job, my registrar tried hard to add to this list by describing the particular expression that patients with peritonism use when asked whether the ambulance journey to hospital was painful: "Only going over the bumps, doc", was to enter the medical literature as Fieldman's sign. Sadly, my column in *Cardiology News* is likely to be its only airing.

"... a detailed knowledge of medical eponyms may be impressive but comes at a price, usually paid during medical finals or higher examinations."

Another example is the typical facial appearance seen in long-standing cigarette smokers; the slightly pale and brawny skin was well recognised some years ago. Unfortunately the author of the article highlighting this phenomenon failed to attach his name to the looks, so now we refer to Marlboro - rather than mitral - facies. Had he instead hailed this observation as Plucknicker's sign (or whatever), we would all be using it in medical notes on a daily basis.

Of the many eponyms that students and trainees might attempt to commit to memory, I would recommend Sutton's law which encourages us to perform the test or therapeutic manoeuvre most likely to establish the diagnosis. An American bank robber in the early 1900s who enjoyed success as well as repeated convictions, Willy Sutton (1901-1980), spent much time behind bars. When once asked by an exasperated judge why he continued to rob banks, he replied, "because that's where the money is".

There seems to be a lack of syndromes, signs or maladies that can be ascribed to contemporary personalities. Perhaps there is little new pathology around. An opportunity to put a surname to HIV infection was clearly missed; perhaps the anticipated avian flu that is about to hit us will provide someone with immortality in the medical textbooks. In cardiology, Brugada is an example, and as new imaging techniques and more sophisticated therapies emerge, there will be further

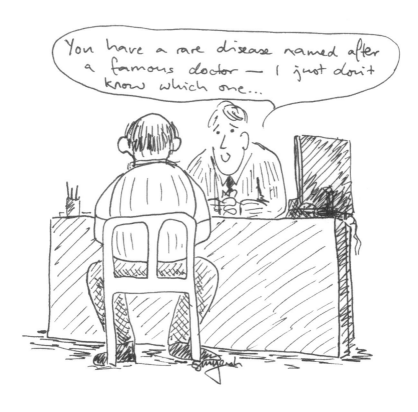

opportunities for quick thinking individuals to get recognition. Even if we fail to settle on an appropriate surname for anatomical structures, we can always describe coronary vascular branches according to the predictable consequence of injudicious catheterisation. Hence, the conus branch of the right coronary is correctly referred to as 'the artery of ventricular fibrillation'.

Given the technological explosion of interventional cardiology it seems odd that this subspecialty has not produced more devices or phrases that are linked to renowned individuals. Aphorisms that guided us in the pre-stent era like "the more you look the worse it gets" (Geoff Hartzler?), or "perfection is the enemy of good" (Richard Myeler?), have sadly gone by unnamed, so perhaps I could offer the following possibilities:

- Norell's sign: if the first spurt of arterial blood from a femoral puncture lands beyond the ipsilateral knee, then the systolic pressure is greater than 180 mm Hg.
- Norell's law: during percutaneous coronary intervention, the patient should never be asked if they have chest pain.
- Norell's dictum: beware the "Triangle of Death" (the cone of tissue at the ostium of a side branch potentially left uncovered when stenting bifurcation disease).
- Norell's triad: never undertake angioplasty on a patient you don't want to treat, who doesn't want treatment, or in whom you cannot see the target lesion.

Having a detailed knowledge of medical eponyms may be impressive but it comes at a price, usually paid during medical finals or higher examinations. We all remember that if we were unwise enough to mention Osler's nodes (after Sir William Osler, Canadian physician, 1849-1919) or Roth spots (Swiss pathologist, 1839-1914) during a viva, the next question we would get was predictable: "And who was ...?"

In obstetrics, final examinations were straightforward as all notable conditions and techniques were named after Swiss-German gynaecologists working at the turn of the nineteenth century. Life was easy ... or was it ... ?

The examiner produced a pair of forceps from under the large mahogany table that separated him from the pale and sweaty obstetric student opposite. "Now, what are these, young man?"

The candidate fumbled with the stainless steel in clammy, trembling hands. "These are obstetric forceps, Sir." The reply was shaky, but nevertheless carried with it a high likelihood of being correct.

"Excellent!" came the encouraging response from the beaming Professor. "And, what are they called?"

From somewhere in the depths of his obstetrics textbook a name popped into his head. "Wrigley's forceps, Sir."

"First class! Well done indeed!" The inquisitor now leant forward, frowned and peered over the top of his glasses and under his bushy eyebrows. "And who was ... Wrigley?"

Fear sapped any moisture from his mouth. The student could feel beads of perspiration developing over his forehead and his abdominal contents seemingly plummeting towards the floor. Then, it came to him. Confidence oozed back into his body like hot chocolate and brandy at the top of a wind swept ski lift. Of course, it's easy! He looked up and cleared his throat as he visualised an Honours viva just around the corner.

"He was a Swiss-German gynaecologist working at the turn of the nineteenth century, Sir", he said with a jaunty air of familiarity.

Silence. Then the creak of wood and leather as the examiner sat back in his chair. A long sigh, as he focused his gaze on the other's eyes. "No, boy. I am Wrigley."

Chapter 2

The ad-man cometh

Traditionally, the medical profession has not excelled in self-publicity. Apart from ethical reservations, perhaps it is also the high esteem and respect bestowed upon us by a grateful public that makes us (well, most of us) reticent when it comes to proclaiming our own successes and that of our departments. One would have thought that, of all specialists, it might be the cardiologist that would be the first to delve into this forbidden arena. Our reputation as aggressive and dynamic, Rambo-esque types, who live life 'in the fast lane', might be deserved in some cases. The more senior readers amongst you may recall the now outdated distinction between the Type A and Type B cardiologist, but this related to their administrative base of operations (tertiary centre and district), not to personality profile.

The modern NHS requires us to poke our heads above the parapet and indulge in some serious self-advertising. If, as we are constantly reminded, our "customers" should be "empowered" to make a "choice" as to where and by whom our "product" is supplied, so that their "journey" and "experience" can be enhanced, then surely - as "providers" - we should be prepared to put out our stall in the market place.

Clinicians rightly sense that the predominant factor in this decision-making should be the quality of care based on a robust infrastructure of audit and clinical governance. But issues such as public transport access, parking, accommodation for relatives and restaurant facilities, have become equally, if not more, important. Whilst we, our managers and clinical coders (the last being a pivotal element in these processes), struggle to produce accurate and meaningful measures of activity and outcome, those more non-clinical factors will continue to be high on the list of considerations when units are compared by patients and carers.

"... advertising in healthcare can be an awkward business and therefore requires a modicum of sensitivity."

Could it be then, that paper doilies on tea trays will be of more concern than enzyme elevations after elective PCI? Hopefully not, but nevertheless we must wise up not only to how our units operate but also to how they are perceived to function (naturally, one assumes that these two measures will be at least similar). Announcing widely that your CCU is open 24 hours a day, is hardly likely to attract patients any more than offering an extra Venflon with every dose of Tirofiban. As with defence contracting and firearms manufacturing, advertising in healthcare can be an awkward business and therefore requires a modicum of sensitivity.

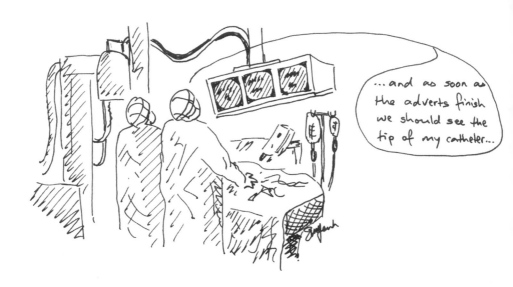

Programmes of public education and health promotion are one thing; commercials advertising medical products are quite another. The age old campaigns around drink-driving and the use of seatbelts ("clunk-click every trip!") are two examples of successful media strategies that are now well established in the public mindset. The gothic horror of collapsing tombstones that warned us of an impending AIDS epidemic and, more recently, images of thick yellow porridge dripping from cigarette ends, may have had more questionable impact.

Alternatively, we are well accustomed to seeing Anadin (or one of a hundred other similar products) as the instant cure for a headache (now, scientifically proven to be caused by arrows entering the neck, rising up to the temples producing 'pressure', then circulating around the forehead and thereby resulting in 'tension'). Typically, UK adverts for conditions between the waist and knees are delightfully coy; a businessman shuffles on a cinema seat, seemingly unable to find relief from troublesome haemorrhoids; a housewife appears puzzled as to how her diarrhoea is going to interfere with the daily programme of school runs, yoga and coffee mornings that lie ahead.

The US approach to such marketing is slick and professional, sometimes bordering on the incredulous. I remember a TV ad-break during CNN when a specific ointment was promoted as being "clinically indicated for PMI*". The accompanying asterisk took my eyes down to the bottom of the screen and its explanation: "Personal Membrane Itch"! Don't Americans have a unique gift for being able to describe literally anything, perfectly?

A particular anxiety of mine - and one of national importance to us - is cardiac pain. How often have we enquired from our infarct patients why they waited three hours at home with their chest discomfort before calling for help? The usual response ("I thought it was only indigestion"), is fascinating, particularly when the patient has had no dyspeptic symptoms before. This misconception is reinforced by a number of TV ads showing a middle-aged man with a painful expression on his face and a hand across the centre of his chest. The reassuring voiceover: "Indigestion? Take Lodabol", perpetuates this mixed message, and the superimposition of bright red and orange flame onto his epigastrium, apparently consuming his torso and licking upwards into his throat, does little to help.

I wonder whether a simpler, more homely message could be produced, perhaps in unsteady, black and white film, or grainy, sepia tones ...

Scene: Bedroom. Camera pans from clock showing 3 a.m. to worried looking gentleman in pyjamas and night cap, sitting up in bed next to sleeping wife (in curlers). Both his hands are flat across his chest.

Morgan Freeman type voiceover: "Central chest discomfort?"

Man looks up at camera and responds with apologetic nod. Wife, now awake, looks at hubby then, earnestly, at camera.

Voice: "Had it before?"

Both parties give anxious looks at each other, then back to camera, shaking heads.

Voice: "Sounds like a possible heart attack. Why, if I were you, I'd get right to it and call for a little ol' ambulance."

They look at each other again, then back to camera nodding in agreement. She reaches for telephone.

Voice: "Oh, and by the way, meantime, why don't y'all take an aspirin?"

Wife nods knowingly, pats husband on head and they both smile.

Fade out.

Chapter 3

"Calm down dear, it's only a vagal reaction"

Recently, I have taken to using a pair of reading glasses. I am advised that I would have needed them sooner if my arms had been shorter, which in a nutshell explains both my golf swing and avoiding ophthalmology as a career. Their ability to transform blurred grey lines into linked words and thereby intelligent or even entertaining communication, is generally accepted. But do not underestimate their far more important function, namely to add emphasis and gravitas (which sounds like a 'serious' political party) to anything you say.

I would recommend you getting hold of a pair - even if they only incorporate just plain glass - and peering over the top of them, while you converse with patients and their families. They seem to take more account of your advice when you sigh that they really should stop smoking, particularly after their third angioplasty, which followed a bypass operation after three documented infarcts. Similarly, nursing staff appear to listen more attentively as you suggest that running wildly down a corridor is probably not necessary, even if the registrar has demanded a litre bag of saline, "NOW!" You will appear pleasantly quizzical as yet another junior doctor refers to "bats wing shadows" on a chest X-ray (oh, really?), or dubious as he tells you of the latest admission who presented with "crushing" central chest pain (did the patient actually use that word?).

As for discussions with managers, I am certain that my spectacles were the only reason we were cleared for 50% drug-eluting stent usage last year. At just the right moment, and having carefully prepared by putting my glasses on the end of my nose five seconds before, I was able to take them off with a flourish and thereby hammer home the point about long-term savings. Holding them between finger and thumb, as I used hand gestures to emphasise that stent prices will fall as more players enter the market, was obviously the clincher.

What one does with reading glasses when not in use, is debatable. You could leave them permanently on the end of your nose, but that detracts from their dramatic value when they are actually required and makes walking down stairs decidedly risky. You could invest in some string, or a similar more fashionable concept, that allows them to dangle harmlessly across the top of your chest (not me, really). Or you could push them northwards to sit above your forehead (my preference). With practice you can then learn to contract certain facial muscles and with an imperceptible nod, the glasses immediately descend to their functioning position. (This is similar to Captain Scarlet's microphone, but never seems to look quite as impressive. It is also less likely to have the same earth-saving results).

My glasses were called upon to fulfil their dramatic function last week when I was informed by our nurse that a patient I had stented an hour before, was back on the ward and had "gone a bit vagal". I contracted the necessary muscles and nodded but the glasses failed to appear on my nose. Having repeated this ludicrous series of twitches twice more without effect, I then remembered that I had left them in my office. Nevertheless, I asked slowly, "What exactly do you mean by vagal?" with my head still positioned as if I had been peering over the rims of my glasses. The predictable answer, "BP seventy, a bit brady and he looks awful", is the nub of today's thesis.

"Perhaps describing a patient as pale, hypotensive and brady-cardic will encourage medical staff to make additional checks as well as calling for the atropine."

We recognise what is meant by a vagal response, usually as a reaction to a noxious stimulus (such as femoral arterial instrumentation), and characterised by pallor, sweating and nausea, followed by bradycardia and hypotension. The management (head down, fluids and atropine) usually works a treat, but thereby reinforces the perception that this is a benign phenomenon and easily treated. I have come across patients in whom the identical syndrome - also described as "vagal" - was (obviously separately) due to a catastrophic upper GI haemorrhage, retroperitoneal bleeding, a femoral arterial haematoma, right coronary artery stent thrombosis and pericardial tamponade secondary to coronary perforation by a guide wire. Whilst each condition may have incorporated a degree of vagal stimulation, the aforementioned treatment might only improve things temporarily. I tend to be concerned that the assumption of an innocent problem that is easily remedied means that the underlying cause of the condition may not be sought and therefore will continue to go unnoticed.

So what is the message as increasing numbers of cardiologists undertake greater volumes of invasive procedures? Maybe we should tell it like it is - not a novel concept, I hope you'll agree - describing clinical situations accurately without presuming the underlying pathology. This might be akin to describing an ECG as showing ST segment depression in leads V1-V3, in preference to simply assuming the presence of anterior wall myocardial ischaemia.

Perhaps describing a patient as pale, hypotensive and bradycardic will encourage medical staff to make additional checks as well as calling for the atropine. As for my reading glasses, their main contribution is time. The second or two required to put them on, or take them off, can provide valuable thinking space. Right now, they're coming off because I feel a bit vagal.

Chapter 4

Teaching cardiology: can we
keep a finger in the pulse?

The recent influx of undergraduates through our Department has meant that I now have a recognised (and importantly, remunerated) session in which to teach.

I have taught students, postgraduates and allied disciplines throughout my career, confident in the assumption that - if not knowledge - then at least my increasing experience would be worthy of passing on to future generations. The results of my endeavours seemed fairly pleasing; I have not been aware of any of my protégés being struck off or imprisoned (at least not for clinical reasons). But like restenosis after PCI, if you don't follow-up you may never know about it.

Unfortunately, the age old aphorism, "see one, do one, teach one", no longer applies. The process of education and training is now appreciated as a complex dynamic, the surface of which - it appears - I have barely scratched. A 'Teaching the Trainers' course, or similar, may be a first step in addressing this deficiency. It throws light on the process and style of educating, and if not addressing the 'what', can certainly give more insight into the 'how'.

The simplicity of cardiology particularly allows medical students to get to grips with the essence of history taking and the rigours of physical examination. We recognise that whilst most of the diagnosis rests on the former, the skills required are by no means easy to pass on. Fortunately there are only four symptoms to worry about (if you are struggling with that, it might be best to stop reading at this point). Emphasising the value of a spontaneous and freely volunteered account of symptoms, contrasts with a continually prompted description of events, interspersed with a random collection of 'yes' and 'nos'. Rule 1: *If you ask questions, all you get is answers.*

We rightly advise caution interpreting terms like 'known case of ...', or the use of quasi-medical terminology, so as to be sure that at least *we* know what is meant by 'palpitation' or 'blackout', even if our patients may not. Looking for a solution like a detective analysing a crime scene, is a commonly used analogy; indeed, the science of deductive reasoning championed by Sherlock Holmes was inspired by a doctor (Joseph Bell) who taught Conan Doyle in Edinburgh Medical School. But extending this to crime movies like "Colombo" is less helpful and thereby brings us to Rule 2: *If a patient looks thoughtful and says, "Doctor, I've just remembered something. This may not be important, but ...", they're quite right; it won't be.*

Medical students sit expectantly in our clinics trying to make a diagnosis on everyone that comes through the door. "Could she have Marfan's?" they tentatively suggest. My response, "I certainly hope not, that's the nurse", seems to disappoint. They look so crestfallen when I warn them that barely 50% of what arrives will have any discernable cardiac pathology. Dedicated chest pain and heart failure clinics are responsible for this, and so we see much more of the 'worried well', and of course, palpitation. Nevertheless, the history remains paramount: "Listen to the patient and he will tell you the diagnosis" is as true today as it always was, whether the individual is well or ill. And so to Rule 3: *The sentence "To be honest, doctor, I feel a bit of a fraud", is to be wholeheartedly welcomed as a reliable and reassuring sign of good health, at least in my experience.*

"The simplicity of cardiology particularly allows medical students to get to grips with the essence of history taking and the rigours of physical examination."

It is unfortunate that cardiac examination has become so engrained into MB BS or MRCP exams. The perception is that the clinical assessment of the heart is commonly undertaken without any background information, which in practice is exceedingly rare. The physical signs are there to point towards, or away from, the possible diagnoses one is already considering based on the history or any other relevant data.

The satisfaction of examining the heart comes from the fact that it's all so tangible. You can see it, feel it or hear it, and if all else fails you can put in a catheter and film it. I was brought up with phonocardiography, M-mode echo, and apex and carotid transducer recordings. Admittedly a full examination took an hour but you really understood the cardiac cycle at the end of it. Trying to enthuse undergraduates with the undeniable logic of a slow rising arterial pulse or reversed splitting of the second heart sound may not be so easy. Sadly, mythology ensures that candidates may still be expected to percuss for cardiac dullness, use a theodolite to locate the apex beat and submit the patient to Kung -fu positions in order to elicit a collapsing brachial pulse. Yet hidden within these rituals lies the essence of the cardiological examination; so, the character of the apical impulse is more important than its location, and of course the same applies to murmurs. Rule 4: *It's more what you hear, and not so much where you hear it.*

The reason we use peculiar hieroglyphics to notate sounds and murmurs is not to separate us from the generality of other physicians, but because we draw what we hear. I became drawn to cardiology when as a registrar I learned from my chief that there were thirteen possible heart sounds. (It's true; when you consider that added sounds and ejection clicks etc., can be left or right-sided in origin, it starts to dawn on you). He used to record not only his auscultatory findings in mitral stenosis with traditional notation, but also indicate the delay between S2 and the opening snap in milliseconds. Surely, we should dissuade our juniors from the ubiquitous "HS I + II + 0" entry into the case notes.

Giving students an idea of what to hear takes imagination. Verbally imitating the quality of murmurs is tricky, but here's a tip. Put the bell of the stethoscope (or more correctly, stethosphone) on your thenar eminence and repeatedly oppose your thumb. You will hear a murmur with the exact pitch and quality of mitral stenosis. Try it.

Chapter 5

Cath lab communication

The development of so many invasive cardiac procedures has required us to function as teams in close proximity. Nowhere is this dynamic more apparent than in the hallowed sanctum of the cardiac catheterisation laboratory and during the practice of PCI. A stethoscope and the ubiquitous half moon spectacles are no longer sufficient for this new role, so what additional skills have we needed to acquire?

We accept the verbal interplay between the lab crew as routine and almost mundane, but to the casual observer - and particularly the patient - the passage of this seemingly bizarre communication can sound complex and even confusing. Thus the phrase "O-ring is open", although seemingly more suited to a gynaecological theatre or lower gastrointestinal procedure, will alert the technician that the sudden drop in blood pressure is the expected consequence of manipulating hardware in the guiding catheter.

The origins of such phrases can be obscure. One of the first live PTCA courses was held in Paris and directed by Richard Meyler who was helped by an extremely able assistant to whom he referred to as "Benny". As the case progressed and the sterile towels over the patient became increasingly bloodstained or sodden with flush and contrast, he would ask his co-operator for yet another coloured drape. Since then, whenever additional protection is required in our lab (and as a mark of respect to the notable jazz enthusiast), the request rings out: "let me have a Benny Green".

The efficient and safe functioning of the lab team is akin to a well trained ship's crew. My interest in sailing and an obsession with the film "Crimson Tide" were both therefore responsible for our trainees watching this film and digesting its contents. PCI then became a perfectly ordered activity with all its procedures, checks and processes running as smoothly as a nuclear weapons test or a torpedo drill. During the more stressful moments (e.g. left main dissection) we even "rigged for ultra-quiet", but stopped short of switching to red light when working during the hours of darkness.

While addressing an LAD lesion, as the guide wire found every single septal branch imaginable, the technician would say "ectopics" to which I would respond "roger that". I have since modified this acknowledgement to "copy that" as occasionally the patient would become concerned that for some reason I was intent on causing untold damage to their coronary circulation.

Similarly, my request for a "three-zero by one-eight Zeta" would be immediately repeated back to me. This would ensure that, 1: it had been heard, 2: it had been understood correctly and 3: to give me the opportunity (not uncommon) to change my mind.

Eventually these procedures were toned down as I increasingly came to resemble Gene Hackman (at least in terms of hairstyle), and we took on a trainee who was the spitting image of Denzel Washington. Nevertheless, I would defend the concept of such an ordered approach, which the following example might illustrate. During a stenting procedure, the question "what is the ACT?" received the response "144". The not unreasonable action was to top up with a further heparin bolus. However, the correct reply should have been "144 *and rising*", the figure eventually settling at 283, not usually indicating the need for more anticoagulation.

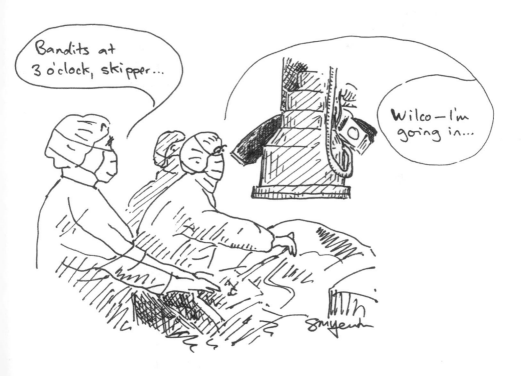

There are of course some things one should never say during PCI, such phrases having the same superstitious significance as naming "The Scottish Play" in The Old Vic. Examples are: "you can call for the next patient now", "I can't remember the last time we sent a case to theatre" and "we should have time for this single vessel chap before lunch".

"Communication between lab personnel should be clear and unambiguous."

Similarly there are certain actions which are either forbidden or should at least be undertaken carefully. I used to work with a colleague in the pre-stent era who, at the end of a case, always removed his gloves slowly and without a sound. He was convinced that the rubbery 'splap' of de-gloving, was somehow able to cause abrupt coronary occlusion. This phenomenon has yet to be tested scientifically.

Communication between lab personnel should be clear and unambiguous. Ideally the operator should direct this verbal traffic, so that if untoward events occur then all know who to turn to for instructions. Similarly it may be preferable for the operator alone to give instructions about moving arms away from the field of view or deep inspiration, otherwise the patient may become confused when he suddenly hears an unrecognisable voice yelling "cough sir, cough!".

Verbal communication is hindered by wearing a theatre mask. Nowadays we have dispensed with these during PCI, which is a good thing unless you are being interviewed by the press. In that case the media almost expect a life-saving cardiologist to be wearing greens (or blues) and have a mask loosely hanging from his neck. This also works very well if you happen to be late arriving for an outpatient clinic.

Professor Bernie Meier, who has been involved with PCI since its inception, has a view on this subject. When performing at live demonstration courses he could converse with a French patient and communicate to a Swiss lab crew, while answering questions from an English speaking audience. To his credit, he also has the sense of humour to match each of these nationalities. He once said that the only reason to wear a mask during PCI was when undertaking laser-assisted angioplasty, and only then so that the patient did not later recognise you.

Chapter 6

"Today we have naming of parts ..."

We prescribe drugs, or ask our scrub nurses for various interventional devices, every day of the week. The requests roll off our tongue like asking for a gin and tonic, or an airline upgrade. Yet do we ever stop to think, "Why on earth (or a similar Anglo-Saxon phrase denoting bemusement) did they call it that?"

Much effort and - more importantly, money - is spent by pharmaceutical companies and the device industry, on the names of their products. Many of us may have attended focus groups when, after refreshments and canapés in a forgettable London hotel, and for what in hindsight was a ludicrously small honorarium, we would give our views on whether "Hear-that-till" was a better name than "What-a-thrill" for the latest converting enzyme inhibitor.

Whilst we just did our best to ensure that our petrol was covered, the management decisions reached after such intense analysis could make a difference of millions to company profits. A memorable and catchy name is ideal, but if it also describes the function of the drug or device, then so much the better. Some examples of the former are engrained in pharmaceutical mythology, such as Nystatin (after N.Y. State Department of Health), Metoprolol (a 'me too' drug) and Lasix (its diuretic effect lasting six hours).

As for interventional cardiology, the imagination required to name the multitude of available equipment, knows no bounds. Naming a guide wire 'The Poker', or a balloon 'The Dilator', is far too simplistic and has been avoided, probably for politically correct reasons. Yet they do accurately describe the purpose.

> "The name of a drug or device may not be the sole determinant of its success in the market, but it undoubtedly plays a part."

Think about it. For a guiding catheter you are looking for a steady, reliable platform, providing predictable support for every case; something like a 'Step-One', 'Base-Camp' or 'Stage-Rite' catheter, sounds perfect. I can hear myself now asking for a 6 French, right Judkins, 'Rock' guide. Guiding catheter diameters have been reduced in order to make percutaneous intervention less invasive but the amount of kit one can then introduce into the coronary circulation becomes limited. One could speculate therefore as to the value of a catheter with an in inner diameter that actually exceeds the outer dimension. Perhaps an internal lining of mirrors would be the secret, and the name 'Tardis' might then be appropriate.

As for guide wires, more subtlety is required. We are now looking to conjure up finesse and sensitivity. We want a one-to-one torque response, variable shaft support, tip angles and strength, and perhaps a hydrophilic coating to find a route through as yet unchartered occlusions. This exploring concept raises the possibility of the 'Cabot',

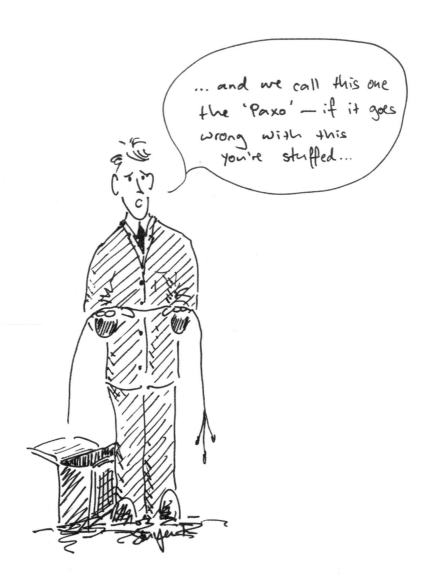

'Magellan' or 'Vasco Da Gama', but instead the 'Pilot', 'Cross-It' and 'Navigator' wires have emerged as more acceptable. There is still something romantic about asking for a 0.014 inch 'Scott' wire, but one could imagine that after hours of trying to cross an impossible lesion, tragedy would supervene and the case would have to be abandoned. To make matters worse, perhaps a Norwegian cardiologist would have already treated the patient successfully.

Promotion goes well beyond simply deciding on a name for a product. When the 'Magnum' wire - featuring an atraumatic olive-shaped tip - was introduced to address chronic total coronary occlusions, one well attended evening launch event was accompanied by the liberal dispersal of chocolate ice creams of the same name.

It is the balloon, however, that has taken marketing departments almost into the realms of Freudian analysis. The final battle between good and evil is represented by pitting man - or rather, balloon - against his nemesis; the monster; his Moriarty; even anti-matter itself: atheroma. This Armageddon-like conflict in the arterial endothelium might equally well take place in the Coliseum, the skies over Kent or the final frontier of space. Hand to hand combat, and the cut and thrust of balloon dilatation, might therefore be expressed in the 'Gladiator', 'Spitfire' or 'Starship Trooper' balloon. It is no coincidence that an 'F14' existed over a decade ago, and the 'Maverick' catheter is in wide use today.

Stenting has required another quantum leap for the imagination of our industry colleagues. The fact that these devices reside permanently in the coronary tree has mandated the need for a careful choice of nomenclature. Something long lasting and steadfast is called for, together with an encouraging hint that its tracking, delivery and deployment will be unproblematic. The 'Vision', 'Liberté' and 'Endeavour' are current players, but historically there were similar examples, although initially their names were not so easy to interpret. A welcome replacement for the original, non-balloon mounted Palmaz-

Schatz stent, was the AVE 'gfx' device. What did that mean? Easy: greater flexibility and crossing!

The name of a drug or device may not be the sole determinant of its success in the market, but it undoubtedly plays a part. I would certainly prefer to ask for a 'Winch', as opposed to a 'Wally' wire, or a 'Spinnaker', rather than a 'Softy' balloon.

The task of choosing a winning name may eventually fall to computers, but I am not optimistic that they will necessarily come to the rescue. Famously, one was used to amass the wealth of marketing information about drug names and sales, and thereby derive what was predicted to be the most successful name, ever, for a cardiovascular agent. Unfortunately it turned out to be 'Cadavaar'.

Chapter 7

Meetings, meetings, meetings

There was I thinking that being a doctor was all about making patients better, but this is only a small part of consultant practice in a tertiary cardiothoracic centre. It is always tempting to spend one's time in the catheter lab, happily crushing stents into yet another bifurcation lesion, while letting the management structure of your hospital continue to grind on without you. However, this is an inadvisable approach, both for side branches and for the functioning of your own unit.

Like it or not we have to take an active part in the running of our departments in order to fight our corner more effectively. Most senior specialist registrars will now include a management course in the ever growing 'Courses Attended' section of their CV, but in general we are still fairly green when it comes to interacting with non-clinical colleagues. Engaging with managers using published data, a clinical evidence base or patient outcomes is all very well, but if what you want to achieve is not on their agenda then you might as well get back to the lab. You have to wrap up and disguise your message so that it appears as a current hot issue and one with which a manager is already grappling, and so will want to hear about. The first thing to do is to learn the language; there is a whole new vocabulary out there and once you tap into it you will be surprised how interesting you become.

Throw in words like 'stakeholders', 'revenue stream' or 'out turn', and eyes light up. Murmur 'commissioning', 'contracts' or 'access rates', and cheeks glow with anticipation. Finally, come out with 'tariff', 'marginal cost' and 'bed stays' and they will become putty in your hands. With their eyes glued on targets, our managers 'scope', or 'do a piece of work' in order to 'understand' door-to-needle times and inter-hospital transfer delays. With thoughtful packaging, the right choice of words and a few well chosen David Brent-type hand gestures, this can present a golden opportunity. Suddenly, and apparently from nowhere, we are asked to ring fence cardiology beds or increase lab sessions which is just what we wanted all along.

Management meetings are an art form and attending them requires careful preparation and training. For maximum effect you should arrive just after the start time and with a large collection of papers under your arm. Of course they will have nothing to do with the meeting at all, but are designed to indicate that you mean business, and also to counteract the enormous diaries in which everyone else is writing continually throughout the proceedings. Ensure that you make some (any) comment - or better still a correction - when going through the minutes of the previous meeting. This signals that you are on the ball and have no intention of letting even the smallest thing escape your attention. A note of caution here; this is inadvisable if you were not actually present.

Sitting just to the right of the chairman is a useful ploy as requests for 'Any Other Business' tend to go clockwise round the table. Your contribution will therefore be at the end, and as by this time everyone is usually exhausted, you may be able to get an item slipped in and accepted without much notice. Finally, when everyone has agreed a date for the next meeting, always come out with a reason why it is no good for you. It emphasises the vital importance of your future presence, is irritating and reminds people that at least you have other things you could be doing.

"Management meetings are an art form and attending them requires careful preparation and training."

Much of the administrative process occurs via e-mail and so an intimate understanding of this technology has become essential. We accept that much of the electronic traffic revolves around missing case notes, a filing cabinet that needs a new home or a desperate need for an inkjet cartridge. Our own system was recently clogged with a heated series of communications about staff car parking. However, somewhere amongst that chaff, are lost vital nuggets of information that require our focused attention. Only then will we avoid discovering one morning that our commissioners will only stump up for one drug-eluting stent this year, and that this had been clearly indicated in an e-mail to which a lack of response was assumed to indicate agreement.

Although it appears to have the informality and immediacy of a phone call, e-mail nevertheless incorporates the permanence of the written word, with all the embarrassing sequelae that this can sometimes bring. Care is always required when deciding casually to 'reply to all' as opposed to just 'reply'. Therefore, the golden rule of letter writing still applies: never send off a letter in haste or anger; always leave it as a draft until the next morning when you can see more clearly just how much of a twit you will appear should the missive actually arrive at its intended destination.

In order to add colour and sparkle to your electronic creations I can thoroughly recommend *Eats Shoots and Leaves* by Lynne Truss, as an entertaining and indispensable guide to correct punctuation.

I have just noticed that the Network meeting which I chair, and in which I am currently penning this article, is coming to an end, thereby bringing this contribution to a natural conclusion. Just before I ask about any other business I shall sign off with this final thought: never put anything in writing and always keep a copy.

Chapter 8

Keeping up with the fluids

Millions of years ago we emerged as basic life forms from the primordial soup, and via the oceans eventually came onto land (well, most of us anyway). Over the ensuing eons our primate ancestors descended from trees and, with thumbs opposed, finally walked erect. It appears, however, that only in the last few years has a basic truth been appreciated; namely the importance of maintaining an adequate water intake.

I am not referring to the vital need for clean drinking water across parched and drought-ridden land masses in the third world, but to the almost religious requirement for liquid in areas where all manner of fluids are already abundant. No work station is now acceptable without an enormous dispenser providing chilled as well as cold water. No self respecting jogger is seen without a plastic bottle ergonomically designed and moulded to be held comfortably in one hand. No secretary's desk would be complete without a two litre bottle of Evian next to her keyboard.

When we appointed some radiographers recently, one of the candidates brought a bottle of water with him into the interview room. Did he anticipate that his questioning was going to take days? Or maybe he thought that our grilling of him was going to be just that: intense and under spotlights!

Perhaps it is global warming or the air-conditioned environments in which many of us work, but apparently we are just not drinking enough. I was reminded of this when I had eventually finished a particularly long morning case, one afternoon. I peeled off the various layers of lead shielding to reveal a sweat-sodden cath lab top. As the only remaining clean scrubs were designed to fit a pigmy, I had no choice but to put up with a damp torso as I made my way to our spacious staff room and a long awaited coffee.

I suspect that it would have been better and certainly more physiological to replace my fluid loss by using the water dispenser. Our labs were specifically designed to have one of these every three yards, so you can't move without stepping over enormous plastic barrels of fresh - and no doubt expensive - drinking water. In addition, in order to ensure that you consume sufficient volumes of liquid, the manufacturers helpfully dispense at least six plastic cups jammed together, rather than the single one actually required. The trouble is that I just didn't *feel* thirsty, and to be honest I think I'm a bit of a coffee nut anyway.

Historically, we have put up with an ancient kettle, milk standing up in the fridge that isn't even in a bottle and a very stained, bent and suspect teaspoon. A mound of brown peculiar smelling powder emerges from a large unlabelled tin and is traditionally referred to as "NHS coffee", although I doubt it has any relationship to either. As one might expect, cath labs on the continent have taken the supply of coffee seriously. In Amsterdam I found fresh espresso available after each case; you could hear the beans being ground as the final angiographic result was documented. I came across the most impressive 'elevenses' during a spell in the Queen Alia Heart Institute in Amman, Jordan. As one would expect in a military hospital, service was prompt and to an exceptionally high standard. The head cardiologist (a brigadier, probably) would mutter a few words to the lab technician, and within seconds a diminutive chap wearing a white tuxedo would appear with a silver tray bearing china cups and fresh Arabic coffee.

"Perhaps it is global warming or the air-conditioned environments in which many of us work, but apparently we are just not drinking enough."

I had significant input into the design 'extras' that went into our new centre. However, although we got live flouro feed from all the labs direct onto multiple flat screens on the wall of our interventionists' lounge (for training and monitoring purposes), I failed dismally to have installed an industrial facility capable of delivering all varieties of authentic fresh coffee, 24 hours a day.

We must remember that caffeine during a list has its disadvantages as well. Granted, it perks you up and brings you rapidly into the 'PCI zone', but it also brings unwanted effects well below the cerebrum that can be problematical, particularly in unexpectedly long cases. Tremor is one example; tying surgical knots with 6/0 Prolene during a Sones procedure is less common nowadays, but threading the back end of a guide wire into the tip of a low profile balloon is hard enough, without the shaking motion equivalent to 6.5 on the Richter scale.

One can take the whole coffee thing too seriously. A colleague has a machine in his office that accepts prepacked pods which, with the addition of hot water (and a squirty sound that resembles someone using a toilet), produces a never ending supply of all types of heart warming beverage. A huge variety of available sachets are therefore stacked in boxes head high on shelves in his office.

But back to water and the basics of life. I am not sure that I - or the more fluid-sensitive components of my physiology - could necessarily cope with consuming the recommended four litres per day. If so, I would have to negotiate another Programmed Activity to allow time to rid myself of the consequences. On a recent ski trip I found myself on a lift with an American businesswoman, whose lavish winter gear was accessorised with a water-containing back pack from which a rubber tube passed over her shoulder to her chin. Apparently it is called a platypus but, like the dodo, I suspect its future on this planet is limited. Although clearly designed to enable effortless drinking whilst on the move, there was one small problem; it was ten below zero and her pipe had frozen.

Chapter 9

Put off by the Ritz

Although I am writing in the height of summer, you will (or should be) reading this when the scorching days of June are long gone. The rhythmic, profoundly irritating and endless series of female grunts that pervaded Wimbledon fortnight, have faded into mere echoes in a distant memory. Henman Hill (now renamed Murray Mound) is deserted for another year, and the 'meetings' season is with us again. This seems to follow two distinct phases; rather than peaks, conference activity is characterised more by its troughs. Cardiological science goes quiet from mid-December and is rejuvenated in the New Year only to retreat into the background again in early July. It is the European Congress in late August that heralds the new beginning of a series of national and international discussions.

Presumably it is the school holiday schedule that produces the template for these arrangements; one conference merging seamlessly into the next, a brief lull for half term, then off again. Preparing power point presentations and posters, attending workshops, chairing sessions and networking with UK colleagues who you only see in foreign climes, is one thing; coping with the increasing complexities of hotel life, is quite another.

It is certainly sad that in many international hotels, the bedrooms, lobby, restaurants or even staff, give no clue as to what country we are in. Cardiologists are well travelled individuals. You would assume therefore that, over the years, we would have become more than familiar with the workings of the Radisson in Delhi, the Hyatt in Dubai or the Hilton in Dorking. Indeed, so familiar that we might even begin to resent the paste on smile of the receptionist who, within seconds of your bedraggled arrival from the airport, requires a credit card for any extras, and asks if you require a newspaper or a wake up call.

And so begins perhaps days of a peculiarly artificial existence that most of us have come to take for granted. We eventually chance upon the lifts which transport us, (together with a small group of oriental air hostesses who I can only presume reside in elevators permanently), to the 15th floor. It is then a ten-minute walk through never ending identical corridors, with bizarrely patterned carpet, until you reach room 1537. You only know this is your assigned room because that is the number on the key card. Now, where's that? Well, you tossed that, along with ticket stubs and other seemingly useless bits of paper, into a waste bin way back when you were in the lobby waiting for the lift.

In and swiftly out with the key card, and after repeated failures signalled by a red light, you sense growing concern that this is indeed the wrong door. Eventually, you realise that the arrow on the card indicates the end to be inserted first. Success! A green light, a buzz and a reassuring click as the door finally unlocks.

The room is impressive. Chilled down to 16 degrees thanks to the 80 decibel air conditioning fan, adorned with the oddest wallpaper and local examples of modern art, and sporting a minimum of two matching king-size beds, each as big as a tennis court. If you were lucky enough to be escorted to your room by a porter, he will brief you as to its contents. He will helpfully indicate the window (the large expanse of glass through which there is a stunning view of an adjacent office block), the TV (the thing that looks like a TV), and the bathroom (the bright white tiled area with two sinks, a shower, a bath, scales, a bidet and two bathrobes - each featuring the hotel's motif - which can be purchased from reception for the equivalent of £55; no wonder people apparently want to nick them!).

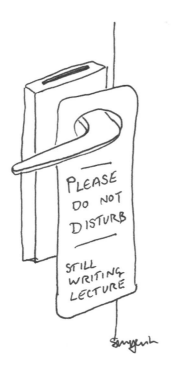

Here also, amongst the conditioning shampoo, bubble bath and covered soap (that cannot be freed from its wrapper without a blow torch), is the now universal advice regarding disposal of towels. In seven languages it pleads with us to prolong the life of our planet by avoiding the need to wash them, and therefore exhorting us to reuse them whenever possible.

"And so begins perhaps days of a peculiarly artificial existence that most of us have come to take for granted."

In an effort to be different from so many near identical chains, the furniture and bathroom appliances are innovatively designed. Unfortunately, by doing so their original purpose was lost sight of long ago. The wash basin is a large square and only three inches deep. After a severe scalding you finally work out how the taps function, and spend the next five minutes locating the plug machinery. Not in this case a lever hidden behind the taps, but a swivelling disc in the middle of the sink. Bending down in a vain attempt to rinse your face, results in you cracking your skull on the edge of a cleverly located glass shelf on which you can find a bowl of cotton wool balls, now handy for dabbing blood from the wound on your forehead.

And so to the minibar. They gave up describing this as an "honour bar" years ago, no doubt because of abuse by the same heartless Venusians who are secretly trying to destroy Earth by carelessly tossing barely used towels into the bath for replacement. A note of caution here: satellite technology can now detect when drinks are taken - even temporarily - from the fridge, so removing the gin bottle and replacing its contents with water, will not work.

Ahhh! A relaxing shower before dinner to sooth away the grime and tension of the six-hour flight. A loud knock produces a hasty egress and shuffling with damp footprints to the door, while wrapped in an enormous bath towel (previously used, of course). Two large, round, Eastern European females, each carrying what look like curtains, greet your drenched face with wide grins and ask whether you require a 'turn down' service. Showing remarkable political aplomb, they interpret your dripping grimace as a "Not now, thank you", rather than the "What the bloody hell are you talking about?" that you intended. No chocolate on your pillow for you tonight, then.

Jet lag, and the drone from the service lift next to your room, results in little if any sleep and therefore you wake, poorly prepared for the most important decision of the new dawn. Should you risk taking your morning ablutions at 6.00 a.m. in the knowledge that you ordered breakfast via room service to be delivered between six and half past? This ludicrously early start was to ensure you caught the once daily bus that will shuttle you (via eleven other hotels), to the Congress Centre 15 miles away.

In due course, after a series of long days, late nights, poor sleep and excessive alcohol, it is checkout time. The lack of any queue when you arrived makes you assume a similar situation when departing. Not so; the lobby is packed with long lines of other miserable attendees, all with the same orange conference bag. They all give anxious glances at their watch, concerned that there is now a high likelihood of missing their flight home.

If only leaving a hotel could require simply a cheery wave. Instead, we are confronted by the same stick-on smile which greeted us three days ago, and interrogated as to whether we dared to use the satellite controlled minibar. Then, just as you thought that the neurons responsible for your sensation of irritation had been down-regulated to have negligible function, comes the final straw. The ultimate reminder that you have been living in a bizarre, parallel universe that bears no relation to normal terrestrial existence: "Would you like your credit card receipt stapled to your bill?"

Chapter 10

Some notes on catheter laboratory atmosphere

The appreciation of background music as an aid to clinical performance is not a new phenomenon. For many years, our cardiac surgical colleagues have been replacing mitral valves to the strains of Beethoven's 6th ("Pastoral") symphony, or perhaps more urgently, repairing post-infarct VSDs to the "Ride of the Walkerie". It was only a matter of time before the new breed of interventional cardiologist realised the benefits of similarly harmonising the atmosphere in the working environment, and thus enhancing the angioplasty experience not only for the operator, but for staff and patient alike.

Industry has certainly appreciated the links between music and interventional cardiology. Examples include the Forté guidewire, and the Solo, Adante and Piccolo balloons. I am assured that a bassoon stent, french horn guiding catheter and Glockenspiel distal protection device are in a developmental stage.

There is not a universal take up of background music amongst interventional operators. Some feel that such 'noise' (sic) represents a distraction and results in underperformance of lab staff. Crucial elements in the PCI procedure may be overlooked; the heparin bolus is forgotten or a systolic pressure of 60 mm Hg goes unrecognised or even ignored until the Monkees "I'm a believer" eventually fades out. The casual visitor to this type of lab environment is immediately struck by the silence and understandably feels the need to speak in hushed tones. Their polite enquiry as to what length of stent the operator plans to use is often greeted by a fierce stare and the muttering of "28" through clenched teeth.

"Much consideration needs to be given to the choice of music. It must suit the mood of the operator but also be at least acceptable to the patient and staff."

Perhaps it is a question of individual comfort. Many have taken on and welcomed the challenges and even tensions that PCI brings. Others may feel these demands have been thrust upon them; they struggle to feel at ease when contrast appears to hang up in the left main stem or, after stent deployment, flow down a large circumflex seems unusually tardy. For the savage beast that lies beneath the modern interventionist, music is guaranteed to provide a soothing influence.

I cannot work in the lab without background music. A silent lab makes me feel that somewhere, something is wrong. If chosen thoughtfully

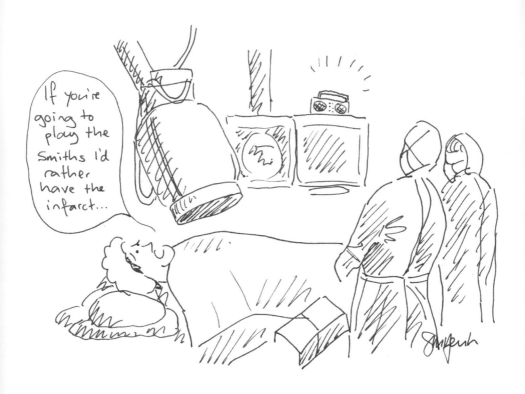

music can provide an efficient working environment in which relaxed staff are still focused on their individual tasks. A quiet lab concerns me; if things begin to go importantly pear-shaped, where then do the assembled staff find the next gear up in concentration. Alternatively, with Nat King Cole wafting around the C-arm, the volume of "Let there be love" can be immediately reduced and I stop singing, thereby indicating to all present that we have now gone to the catheter lab equivalent of DEFCON 3.

Much consideration needs to be given to the choice of music. It must suit the mood of the operator but also be at least acceptable to the patient and staff (this might exclude the latest offering from "Limp Biscuit"). It must truly be in the 'background' and not dominate the lab. I realised the importance of this when I once noticed the movements of my guide wire and balloon were alarmingly in time with Elton John's "Don't go breaking my heart". Familiarity is the key so as to avoid the need to struggle to hear lyrics, or concentrate on following a complicated refrain. Whether one chooses songs or instrumentals is a question of personal preference; as in many other areas of PCI, there is a paucity of randomised data available here.

My selections are exceedingly varied and I cannot explain the basis for a particular choice on a particular day, or for that matter even for a particular lesion subset. Superstition has played a part; when we were recruiting into the Stent Or Surgery (SOS) trial, patients randomised to PCI were fortunate enough not only to receive stents, but also to be soothed with the many and varied hits from our lab's "ABBA Gold Selection". The requirement for Gene Pitney's "24 hours from Tulsa" in order to address an ostial diagonal lesion is less obvious.

I have recently been taken with a string of 60s and 70s hits. Nostalgia may play a part but patients also seem to enjoy these, probably reflecting the fact that I am now treating more patients of my own generation. The more youthful cath lab staff remain bemused, unable to understand the joy with which I and the patient correctly time the bullwhip inserts in Dave Dee, Dozy, Beaky, Mick and Titch's "Xanadu" or that solo drum insert in Phil Collins' "In the air tonight". Commonly, anything by Dean Martin, Frank Sinatra, Bryan Ferry or the Shadows, is more than acceptable to all parties.

Opera can be unpredictable as Antonio Colombo aptly demonstrated at a TCT meeting in Washington a few years ago. Whilst he was undertaking DCA, the patient who himself was a professional opera singer, suddenly burst into song accompanied by a classical guitarist who was also in the lab. I too cannot help singing along with the more memorable arias, only a smattering of Italian and ignorance of the words proving little in the way of a hindrance.

One has to respect the alternative view and acknowledge that to some the only bars heard in the lab should be those referring to the balloon inflation pressure. On the other hand I remain committed to the soothing relaxed but focused atmosphere that cath lab music brings. As for a favourite choice, I am taken by Albert Fennech's consummate guidance in this area. Late of the Brooke Hospital and now a Professor of Cardiology in Malta, he used to encourage patients to bring their own musical tastes with them. I got caught out badly with this arrangement and had to struggle through a long multivessel case with nothing but the sound of panpipes for audio company. A Richard Clayderman selection should probably be avoided in similar circumstances. Prof. Fennech's advice to patients, however, provides the necessary degree of security: "You can bring in anything as long as it's not Country and Western."

Chapter 11

"No dilatation without representation"

"I wonder whether you've tried our latest guide wire?" The hopeful voice of the attractive young lady on the other side of the lead glass partition trails off, then to be lost below the whine of the generator which accompanies the next acquisition run.

I smile apologetically and reply above the hum of the machinery, and the ever present background tones of Nat King Cole: "I don't think this chronic occlusion is going to be straightforward so I'd rather use something more familiar. Perhaps we could chat later?"

Representatives from the device industry have become commonplace in the catheter lab and play a pivotal role in the interventional environment. Some of these individuals have been in the business since angioplasty first took off in the UK. Over the subsequent 25 years they may have changed their allegiance as various companies have combined with others, been swallowed up by larger fish or just fell by the way side, their one and only product never really finding its ideal niche in the percutaneous management of coronary disease. Nevertheless, their enthusiasm and resilience knows no limits. They remain a knowledgeable resource and in some cases have become trusted colleagues or valued friends.

But how do we balance our relationship with industry, particularly with ever increasing management - not to mention media - scrutiny? What do we want, or need, from that interaction and what if anything can we do for them (apart from buying their devices, of course)?

My youthful foray into this area was as a registrar attending occasional pharmaceutical soirees when I and my contemporaries would give apparently valued opinions on the proposed marketing strategies of upcoming drugs. I am reasonably confident that my own contribution to these focus groups (as they are now called) was unlikely to be responsible for any subsequent clinical or financial disaster.

"Representatives from the device industry have become commonplace in the catheter lab and play a pivotal role ..."

Financial assistance to attend and present at, international meetings, was followed by support of the Junior Cardiac Club. Largely, but not exclusively London-based, this society allowed cardiologists in training to get together and share experiences. We would gossip, swap notes, moan about yet another unsuccessful recent interview, practice upcoming presentations to a critical audience and sample a taste of what life might be like in the rarefied atmosphere of a consultant post.

Regular evening meetings, hosted in rotation at various London hospitals, were enthusiastically sponsored, as was dinner afterwards.

International conferences were also arranged, particularly to incorporate non-UK speakers, thereby justifying venues like Reykjavik, Cologne, Portofino and naturally, Grindelwald. It was during a debate in the late 1980s, at one such a meeting in the Bernese Oberland, that I managed to persuade the JCC that patients with acute myocardial infarction were best managed only with "oxygen, morphine and a sympathetic nurse", rather than thrombolytic therapy - for which the available evidence was then, to say the least, compelling and which was then emerging as a major advance in infarct treatment. (I feel this more than demonstrated the open mindedness of our society, although I accept it might have cast a shadow over the quality of the next generation of senior colleagues).

The balance between the academic sessions (7.30 a.m. till 10.00 a.m. then 4.00 p.m. till 7.00 p.m.), and social/recreational activities undertaken in the intervening period, was stringent and acceptable to all parties; it continues to be a successful template for current Alpine-based conferences - apparently. The extent to which the device and pharmaceutical industry support education and training cannot be underestimated. A Trust's budget for staff training or study leave would be rapidly depleted if commercial support or sponsorship was not available.

But what of the one-to-one interaction with company representatives? How is this two-way process best managed? I used to give presentations to industry about how to get the most from this association. I stressed the importance of simply showing interest in an interventional procedure, rather than being glued to their mobile phone arranging the next appointment, and regardless of whether or not their company's stent was to be used.

They should know their product backwards: guide catheter and wire compatibility, stent strut thickness, percentage recoil and shortening, nominal deployment pressure, expansion diameter at every known balloon pressure and metal-to-artery ratio.

They must respond to the question, "What is the crossing profile of this then?" without a split second's hesitation. "Oh-three-two of an inch", they should snap back, as I roll the tip of the device thoughtfully between finger and thumb. When I look at them doubtfully, and suggest, "It feels more like oh-three-three?" they should not look aghast, feeling that they have been caught out or let down by their manufacturers, but simply wait for the smile that follows.

What of the "what not to do"? Well, never say to an interventional cardiologist that he (it is usually a male issue) should use a device because "Ricky Bigballs, at the newly established, 200 case per year, Nether-on-the-Wapping PCI unit, likes it and uses it all the time". Why? Three reasons: 1. he/she probably does not know him well enough to use his first name; 2. it is highly unlikely that he does use it all the time, and only said this to shut him/her up; and 3. the last reason I would use it would be that Dr. Bigballs (for whom I have little time) recommended it anyway.

And don't add, "And he's bought twenty of them", because my personal - and often used - response will be, "Well you won't need me to buy any then, will you?"

On a behavioural note, I am informed that when we interact with company representatives, it is considered to be a successful 'hit' if, during the conversation, we somehow find ourselves mentioning the product in question at least three times. Furthermore, the universal default strategy of terminating a discussion (i.e. doctor stands up), will not work in this setting as our visitors are trained (no doubt in a Pavlovian fashion) to ignore such clear, non-verbal communication.

Industry looks to us for an invaluable clinical perspective and an occasional reality check. Our input into their focus groups or advisory boards is of vital importance ensuring that they do not invest huge amounts of time (or money) going down a fruitless or unnecessary research programme or marketing strategy. This explains the absence of my own potentially valuable and innovative interventional tools from the current device armamentarium. Alas! The 'Wiggle Wire', 'Polo Neck Stent' and 'Norelli Balloon', never saw the light of day.

I am unsure as to the value of so called 'detail aids', those laminated file-bound pages of bar charts, graphs and tables showing the advantages of this or that device over its competitors. I would be concerned if I relied on visitors for information that I should already know. On the other hand I do value the information they provide in terms of upcoming meetings, technical advice and of course, gossip. What are other units up to? One not only learns about a distant lab being shut down because of fire or plague, or tragic events that may have befallen an unfortunate colleague; more importantly you hear news about yourself. I was intrigued to learn recently that not only had I applied for various jobs elsewhere but also that I had even been appointed!

Representatives are one of the few outside individuals that have access to the innermost workings of multiple organisations. They are the bees that hover from flower to flower and thereby receive or donate snippets of information. Particles of data-laden pollen are picked up and deposited, thereby providing knowledge, news, support, entertainment and, occasionally, a kernel of information from which yet another urban myth may grow. Life would be the duller without them.

Which reminds me, I have a new guide wire to look at ...

Chapter 12

That's entertainment!

Unusually, I found myself watching an episode of "Casualty" last week. Or perhaps it was "Holby City", or maybe "The Golden Hour". Anyway, there were certainly some pretty ill people, as well as a plethora of medical staff, nurses, porters, social workers, trolleys and perhaps a helicopter.

The pace was frenetic. It was seemingly impossible to keep up with just who was having the subarachnoid haemorrhage, which of the elderly patients was hypothermic and where that drug addict was who had secretly entered the hospital for a purpose other than visiting his sick granny. And then there was that ghastly looking young chap in the cubicle with the perfect marriage, young family and promising career, who apparently had been as fit as a flea until yesterday. Who was going to tell him the cause of his acute abdominal pain was a high grade, disseminated cancer with a prognosis that was likely to coincide with the closing credits?

It is a long time since I was exposed to the 'frontline' of the A/E department, so perhaps those experiences are a little hazy. But I cannot recall many clapped out patients that came into the resuscitation room and were greeted by someone who had clearly just stepped from the front pages of Vogue magazine. In less than five seconds, she has inspected, palpated, percussed and auscultated all known bodily systems. With one succinct question, "Is that painful?" (answer: a grunt), she goes into action immediately with a practised air of calm authority.

"I want an ECG, FBC, ESR, profile and sugar. Let's tube and bag him, give me three large bore IVs and an 'A' line. Cross match for ten units of 'O-Neg' and organise X-rays of his pelvis, spine, skull and right ankle. Hold three theatres, get me the vascular, neuro and gynae registrars, and get a CAT scan of his abdo and thorax." She adds "Stat!" as an afterthought just in case the urgency of the moment had been lost on the assembled staff.

Speed, of course, is of the essence as the whole case has to be diagnosed, treated and either discharged home or undergo autopsy (with a result), within the next forty minutes. As much as I too would have loved to treat infarct-related ventricular premature beats by yelling, "OK, people! Gimme me 500 of lido in half a bag of D-5-dubbya", I never really got the chance, and anyway no one would have understood what I was talking about.

Do we watch medical dramas and think to ourselves: "Hold on, it just never happens like that"? Somewhere along the line reality has given way to entertainment, rather than education. Instead of standard texts, I must confess that most of my knowledge of pathology was derived from numerous episodes of "Quincy, M.E.". Indeed this energetic coroner spread himself across so many other specialities - psychiatry, obstetrics, social work - I think I could have confined myself to afternoon TV rather than attend medical school at all. I was particularly taken with the sense of urgency with which he exhorted his oriental assistant to, "Rush this through the lab, Sam". To run around pleading for immediate access to various life-saving procedures when a desperate patient is on the brink of expiring is one thing, but when the victim is already showing evidence of *rigor mortis*, this does seem a tad unnecessary. But, heck! It was riveting stuff!

"Somewhere along the line reality has given way to entertainment, rather than education."

The factual accuracy portrayed in these series is impressive; no one should doubt the quality of the medical advice behind each episode. But it is the way in which every possible life event is compressed into such a limited time frame that leaves one aghast. Thirty years ago, my father (a GP) helped with a BBC drama series set in a North London surgery. Called, imaginatively "The Doctors", I guess it was a contemporary version of Dr. Findlay's Casebook (I fear I may be losing more junior readers at this point). He was forever despairing that the script writers/director would want to manufacture much more absorbing and attractive TV material than could possibly be contained in day to day, mundane family medicine. What those with medical knowledge find interesting or even fascinating, falls far short from that required to whet the appetite of the watching, lay public.

As a result, a routine - or even busy - A/E shift has to be 'sexed up' to give it the required general appeal; relationships between the characters become not so much complicated as down right incestuous. So the young lady admitted with the threatened miscarriage turns out to be the partner of the hospital anaesthetist as well as the daughter of the

Casualty consultant who is the ex-husband of the department manager who is now married to the Chief Executive (are you still following this?) who is having an affair with the senior sister who is pregnant but unsure of the father who is actually a junior doctor who was originally going out with the girl who came in at the beginning of this paragraph.

This exaggeration of life cannot just be confined to healthcare-related programmes; I assume that the same yawning gap between reality and TV/film applies similarly to past episodes of "Dixon of Dock Green" or more recently, to "Judge John Deed". I can imagine an off duty Detective Inspector being equally bemused as he watches the totality of police life unfolding into a succinct, hour long "The Bill" special.

So if you thought you might at least get an idea of other professions by watching their representative TV series, I would not be optimistic. Forensic medicine may not be quite as lively as portrayed in "Waking the Dead" or "CSI Miami". And if you fancied yourself as an undercover operative indulging in the odd 'black op' or a touch of espionage, I would not look to "Spooks" to give you the necessary background either. Truth may be stranger than fiction but, sadly, it is just not as entertaining; reality does not come along in neatly packaged sound/vision bites to fit our ever decreasing attention spans.

Right! Where's the TV? I've got to get back to Casualty. Apparently a guy has just gone into his local hospital with a virus that, if released, could destroy all life as we know it on this planet - and they've only got twenty minutes to sort him out. "I want an MSU for M, C & S, sputum and swabs of all orifices. Give me some Strepsils and get micro on the blower ... NOW!"

Chapter 13

"Never forget that you have a choice"

While we all grapple with the increasing absurdities of political correctness, 2006 has brought with it another 'PC' of equally baffling proportions. Yes; as promised, patient choice is with us. How arrogant to think that five years at a medical school, and perhaps another ten at the clinical coalface, could mean that - as even many of our patients suggest - "doctor knows best".

We embrace a patient-centred (rather than a patient-led) NHS but even so, when our patients are offered options the majority will simply say, "what ever you recommend". They perhaps rightly assume that we have considered the various options pertinent to their care and, with their best interests in mind, are now in a position to offer an opinion. They patently rely on what has always been the foundation of the doctor-patient relationship - namely, trust. (Oddly, those words 'foundation' and 'trust' still have pride of place in the modern NHS, but in an altogether different context).

Look ahead to 2010; what will cardiac care be like five years from now?

"We embrace a patient-centred (rather than a patient-led) NHS but even so, when our patients are offered options the majority will simply say, 'whatever you recommend'."

A tie-less, nineteen year-old, senior primary care physician seeks to 'purchase' a coronary revascularisation procedure from the nationwide chain of Tescos Cardiothoracic Centres, and dials their generic 0800 number ...

"Welcome to the Cardiac Procedures Choice Helpline!

"In order to help us process your choice needs we have introduced a series of numbered options which will take you through our range of cardiological and cardiac surgical care products. Your selection from our numerous menu possibilities can be made from the keypad of your phone, as well as by using our speech recognition system. In order to maximise the customer experience of this system please ensure that you speak slowly and clearly into the mouthpiece of your telephone handset when prompted by the tone [Beeeep].

"So that we can ensure equity of healthcare access throughout the United Kingdom our speech recognition software is designed to respond to all regional accents and dialects, as well as voice requests and

commands from a full range of ethnic minorities. We apologise if your dialect or ethnic minority accent is not recognised; if you have difficulty in using our system please refer to the Oxford Glossary of English Language Pronunciation for further help.

"If your client has single vessel disease, press 1, for two-vessel disease, press 2, for three-vessel disease, press 3, and for left main stem disease, press 4.

"Thank you. You have reached the [robotic voice] - 'coronary revascularisation menu'. If your client requires revascularisation for symptomatic relief, press 1. If your client requires treatment to improve his or her prognosis, press 2. If treatment is required for both symptoms and prognosis, press 3. If you wish to hear these options again, press 4, or press the star key at any time to return to the main menu.

"Thank you for choosing [robotic voice again] - 'revascularisation for symptomatic and prognostic benefit'. In order to access your preferred mode of revascularisation, please select from the following three options. Press 1 for coronary artery bypass grafting, 2 for percutaneous coronary intervention or 3 for a hybrid procedure.

"You have chosen CABG on symptomatic and prognostic grounds. We now need to take you through our comorbidity and Euroscore checklist. Please key in your client's age in years. Thank you. Now please key in the latest serum creatinine level in millimoles per litre. Thank you. If the left ventricular ejection fraction is less than 30%, press 1; if there is significant lung disease, press 2; if there is significant peripheral vascular disease or neurological deficit, press 3. If your client has more than one of these options, please press 4.

"Thank you. We now need to assess the urgency of your selected revascularisation procedure. If the surgery is to be routine, press 1; if there has been a recent period of instability, acute coronary syndrome or myocardial infarction in the last six weeks, press 2; if there are ongoing symptoms at rest, fluctuating ST segment changes or haemodynamic compromise, press 3; if your client is in extremis, or is currently receiving external cardiac massage, please press 4 to return to the main menu and then press the star key to access our religious and alternative belief systems selection.

"I'm sorry. We are unable to offer CABG for prognostic benefit in this client because of [pause, robotic voice yet again] - 'increased surgical risk resulting from: age over 80, poor lung function, renal disease, no available conduits, previous stroke and salvage procedure'. Please return to the main menu for alternative revascularisation options ...

"Welcome to the PCI Patient Choice Helpline!

"We are sorry but we are unable to offer PCI for prognostic benefit at this time because of [robot, this time a little like Stephen Hawkin's voice synthesiser] 'lack of Class 1 indication and/or level A evidence base'. Would you like to consider PCI for symptom relief? [Beeeep]. Thank you. You have selected [robot], 'PCI for symptom relief'.

"Would you like your chosen PCI procedure to be undertaken via the radial or femoral approach? [Beeeep]. I'm sorry. I did not understand your response. Did you want a radial or femoral approach? [Beeeep]. I'm sorry. Our system is having difficulty recognising your request for the site of arterial access required for your selected health enhancement option. Please speak slowly and clearly into your telephone mouthpiece. If you require help in pronunciation please access the OED website on www.speakproper.com. Now, for the third time, radial or femoral? Thank you. [Almost imperceptible sigh].

"Now, please key in the number of target lesions to be treated. Thank you. You may now select from our extensive range of diagnostic or therapeutic device options. Press 1 for quantitative coronary angiography, intravascular ultrasound or pressure wire evaluation; press

2 for thrombus extraction or removal, rotational, directional atherectomy or distal embolism protection; press 3 for Reopro or other adjunctive pharmacology; or press 4 to just slam-dunk the lesion with a stent.

"Thank you. Now, please indicate the specific type of drug-eluting stent you require. [Beeeep]. You have asked for [pause] - peanut butter. Did you mean [pause] - Paclitaxel? [Beeeep]. Thank you. Now please key in the reference diameter of the target vessel in millimetres. Thank you. Now, please key in the length of the target lesion in millimetres. Thank you.

"I'm sorry. We are unable to offer you a drug-eluting stent for this lesion on this occasion because [pause, Stephen Hawkin] - 'it does not comply with NICE Technology Appraisal No. 71, published 2003. Please press 1 to select from our bare metal stent options, or hold for an advisor ...'

Bland guitar music, the melody of which appears to go round and round with no discernable start or finish ...

10 minutes later ...

"Welcome to the Cardiac Procedures Choice Helpline!"

Chapter 14

Do you know your number?

I was sitting on the M1 last week (in a car, obviously) held up because of lane closures, a pile up, barrier repairs, shear volume of traffic, an 'incident', a body found underneath a bridge, or possibly all of these. Alternatively, I suspect that two lanes had been coned off for four miles in order to allow a team from the Highway Agency sufficient safe working space to clear a cigarette packet that had strayed dangerously near the central reservation during a recent gusty spell.

The stretch of tarmac between Northampton and Milton Keynes is not noted for its stunning views, so my attention was largely - if not entirely - fixed on the number plate of the sad, silver (originally), Mercedes that sat in front of my bonnet at varying distances, depending on how enthusiastic I was about keeping up with the vehicular flow. And it got me thinking ...

Car owners are divided into those that don't give a hoot (or parp?) about their vehicle registration number, and a small but increasing proportion who spend much energy, time and money in personalising the 5 by 24 inch, plastic strips that adorn each end of their beloved motors. I know for a fact that cardiologists (well, at least one) are not immune from this obsession. Is this simply a reflection of the nature of the beast - the need to be individual, yearning to be different, striving to stand out from the crowd? Or is it that the specialty itself is so riddled with three letter abbreviations that it provides the perfect medium in which to express that which is quintessentially 'us'? (I suspect that you are now beginning to appreciate just how long this queue of traffic actually was).

I am not so interested in the use of one's initials, although I appreciate that this still says something about the owner - perhaps that he is prone to forgetting his name. I am more intrigued with the use of cardiological terms, and thereby the range of possibilities that present themselves to the more imaginative and committed car owning heart specialist.

The trick is to avoid making them so obscure that you have to explain your particular alphanumeric combination to everyone - well at least to those who, for some unfortunate reason, made the mistake of asking you whether the LVH, AMI, or LAD that adorn the fore and aft of your Volvo, might conceivably have some sort of circulatory connotation. (ECG is easy because it is appreciated by colleagues and patients).

Getting hold of the right plate used to attract a degree of cache. It might have taken years to track down the perfect item through the small ads and the Sunday papers, and then to negotiate a price for the car that you didn't really want, but that was usually attached. There could be a major cross country trek in order to acquire your prize, depending on the specific letter combination which originally denoted the region in the UK where the car was registered. (As MSN was of Scottish origin I chose not to bother with that).

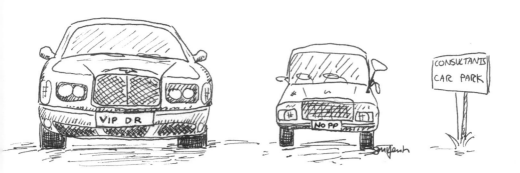

Nowadays, there's nothing to it! The DVLA have twigged that there is revenue to be gleaned by retaining, and later selling off at higher prices, certain attractive combinations. If the plate is available, price depends on whether the year is current, with the single digit '1' being most expensive, 2 to 9 less, and double or treble figures, least. (My offer to the Licensing Authority with specialist advice as to which letter assortments would be particularly suited to my colleagues, has thus far been ignored). Nevertheless, the following paragraphs might provide some examples.

JVP, EDP and (forgive me) VPB, are straightforward enough. It starts to get more demanding when the letters sit alongside various numerals. The recent need to incorporate a two letter prefix now allows many more exciting possibilities. I think that G0 4 PCI is quite clever, and certainly less concerning than A1 4 VF. For the clinical pharmacologists amongst you, I might suggest H1 BP or L1 PID, whilst those who hanker after traditional bedside teaching might prefer S1 LUB, S2 DUP or even 316 ESM (think about it).

A cardiac surgeon who excels in valve repair could consider P3 MVR, but the degree of expertise required to follow the thought processes involved are likely to overwhelm his colleagues, as well as most of you. There is little to be gained from being so obtuse that only you appreciate the thinking behind such a sequence. So, if to understand the reasoning underlying T39 SBE, one requires a copy of the Da Vinci Code, I would suggest getting a bike instead.

"I suspect that one of the reasons we want to stamp our own mark, is to resist the ever increasing tendency for so many facets of our lives to be distilled down to a series of letters or numerals."

And why shouldn't patients share in this immensely satisfying experience? A heart failure patient on excessive diuretic therapy might helpfully remind their physician with K3 LOW, whilst one who is being followed up with aortic stenosis should have AVG 40 (with instructions to change this annually, of course). DUN 4 would best be avoided.

But what to do when the car itself has outlived its usefulness? Well, clearly the registration can be transferred onto the incoming replacement, or advertised to another cardiological colleague (in the back pages of the *Br J Cardiol*, perhaps?). Otherwise it may still be possible to make your own letters just as interesting, even to a non-cardiac customer. I used to have a Triumph Spitfire with NNV (Northampton, by the way) on the plate. Back in London, and to assist its sale, I scoured the phone directory for a suitable name with an address in reasonable proximity. For three weeks my gleaming car, sporting a huge 'For Sale' notice, sat proudly outside the home of a Mr. Nigel N. Vanhorn of Maida Vale, West London. (Simple modesty - and the small matter of truth - does not allow me to report a total success with this ploy, but you get the idea).

I suspect that one of the reasons we want to stamp our own mark, is to resist the ever increasing tendency for so many facets of our lives to be distilled down to a series of letters or numerals. It was Patrick Magohan as "The Prisoner", who said famously, "I am not a number, I am a free man". We should strive to maintain our individuality in this alphanumeric world. (That second bit wasn't him; it was me). That is why I am quite taken with American adverts in which companies give their phone numbers often as catchy phrases. They remind us to, "Touch 0800 HEART-DOC for all your cardiac concerns". British Gas might more truthfully use 0870 WAIT-4-EVER, and as for my bank, I suspect 0845 DONT-BOTHER would be most appropriate.

Telephone numbers used to incorporate a three letter prefix which identified the local exchange. There was something quaint and romantic about giving your number as TUDor 3656 or HIGhgate 3979, while MAYfair 872 or BELgravia 3841 would certainly raise the odd eyebrow. I do wonder whether WHItehall 1212 will still get you through to Scotland Yard, (and perhaps - as in the long forgotten TV police series "No Hiding Place" - directly to the right ear of Detective Chief Superintendent Lockhart).

Well, the M1 has not improved. Today, I suspect a car fire or a jack-knifed lorry at Junction 13 which is responsible for me having been stationary for the last two hours. It has, however, allowed me to write this piece on my laptop, and take more than a passing interest in the blue Peugeot in front. A nodding wife in the passenger seat, a nodding Alsatian on the back shelf, and an apposite number plate which, coincidentally, I can now use ... B1 4 NOW.

Chapter 15

This sporting life

Nursing an injured knee, I have had no choice recently but to become more of a spectator - rather than a partaker - of any form of competitive physical activity. This has meant putting on hold jogging, skiing, occasional tennis and even rarer, golf. Sadly, it has not avoided standing for hours in a catheter lab, covered in lead and treating long segments of diffuse coronary disease by ingeniously reconstructing vessels with many millimetres of stainless steel.

Predictably, this has been frustrating. Nevertheless it has allowed more time to contemplate what similarities may exist between modern cardiological practice and the popular sporting world, as brought to us particularly by television and radio.

Discussing an upcoming challenge, its anticipated difficulties and how they are to be overcome, applies to both environments. A ruddy faced, gum chewing, football manager, with a reputation of being the human equivalent to the Mistral, assures us that the Chelsea strikers will be thwarted by his back four dropping deep (where is that exactly?) and using more width. Similarly, our colleagues (some of whom specialise in making simple angioplasty, complex) describe how two sequential trifurcation lesions will be addressed using a 9 French guiding catheter, six wires and sufficient simultaneous balloon/stent action to be described as, not so much a 'kiss', as an orgy.

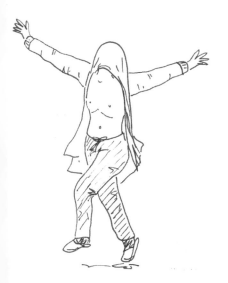

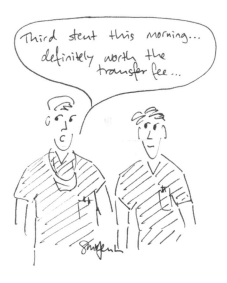

At the time of writing, the winter Olympics have begun in Turin and our TV screens are dominated by a bizarre montage of ice dancing, curling, speed skating (clearly a body hugging Lycra suit is essential here), and of course - luge. How an Olympic event could ever have been devised as to require simultaneous cross country skiing and intermittent rifle shooting, has never been explained. It begs the question as to why mogul skiing and figure skating have never been combined. (Oh! I've just learned - apparently they have).

I am not so sure that the commentators are as clued up as we think either. They keep up their usual monologue during the mens' downhill ... "Schultz then, from Austria, only 19 years of age, going out wide on the Sharpen-Cornen; he won't be happy with that!".

Or ... "And Wolfang Gluber - so clever at downhill that he is known as 'the fox', is going very well indeed. This is fast!" Surely with such small time differences separating the top performers, the only way David Vine can tell that A is going faster than B, is that the split time on his (and our) screen, is 0.001 seconds better.

"They yak the yak, but can they crack the plak?"

It is undoubtedly the 'post-event' debriefing that fails any reasonable expectation of contributing to the overall sum of human knowledge. Given the reported salaries of some individuals we perhaps wrongly anticipate a bit more 'depth' - for instance, from a Formula One driver (who, let's face it, if he's got any sense, tries to go as fast as he can by putting his foot down), or a golfer (objective: get the ball in the hole in as few strokes as possible). Tennis players are the most disappointing; "When he broke me at 4:3, I knew I had to work hard (surprise!). I've been practising my serve (good idea), and my ground strokes (good idea too, whatever they are), and I think that paid off." One is left only wondering who can don the most ridiculously designed baseball cap so that at least the sponsors will get something out of the after-match TV interview.

What might be the interventional cardiological equivalent of such earth-shattering revelations? We listen with caution to those who 'talk the talk', awaiting confirmation that they can also 'walk the walk'. In angioplasty parlance, the equivalent adage has become: "They yak the yak, but can they crack the plak?"

Scene: a sweat-soaked interventionist - his sterile gown bloody and undone - stands in front of a hoarding sporting various device company logos. No sooner has the Angioseal been deployed, than the interviewer steps forward and begins his interrogation.

"Well, Doctor, that certainly looked like hard work. I imagine you're pleased with the final result?"

"Yes. I knew that the combination of calcification, small calibre and diffuse disease was going to make it difficult. I had done a left main bifurcation last week so I knew what to expect."

"Were you concerned when the right went down? Given his poor LV, he didn't tolerate it very well. What did you say to your assistant half way through?"

"Well, obviously we had to reopen the right in a hurry, but it certainly looked better with the seven stents." (He wipes a speck of blood from his cheek and signs a drug chart thrust under his nose). "We talked about how we should approach the left and made some changes; in particular, the balloon pump went in."

"It really was a case of three vessels. Did you feel that bringing out the Rotablator for the LAD proved to be a decisive moment?"

"Definitely; it really made the difference, and upsizing to 8 French as well gave us more options in the left main. After that the circumflex was straightforward with direct stents into each of the two marginals."

"You've got a bit of a break now to prepare for your next case. Are you going to make any changes?"

"Well, my trainee has got to go to clinic, so I'll be scrubbing with our staff nurse. We've got a graft case next so we'll switch the Rotablator for distal protection. Our covered stents have been suspended, so we'll go with a Filter Wire instead."

"Well, good luck with that! I'm sure you'll be relieved with the outcome of that last case given the widespread publication of individuals' results, together with your recent blip?"

"Sure. We know that Dr. Foster is just around the corner but given adjustment for pre-procedural risk, I'm not too worried. Our surgeons had already turned him down so this was always going to be a tricky one. It really is a question of taking each case at a time." He smiles, holding up a used balloon in one hand and a filter wire in the other. Unfortunately the cameraman cannot focus sufficiently quickly to show the maker's name or logo, so a major commercial opportunity is lost.

"Thanks for your time, doc, and with that, back to the ward."

Such a seemingly bizarre scenario is not such a long way off; the panel or 'faculty' discussion so often seen during live or recorded cases, is in a similar vein. The only item missing might be a "Spot the Stent" competition, when the audience are asked to put crosses on an angiogram identifying the proximal and distal ends of the implanted device.

Well, it's time for my knee to get some physiotherapy while I sit back and watch the ski jumping. You've got to be impressed; it is not enough to throw yourself into the air with two large planks on your feet, land with slyle and then come to an eventual stop without decimating the gathered spectators - you have also got to remember to remove one of your skis and hold them up so that the maker's name is plainly visible. Now, I wonder if he could do that and stent the left main stem at the same time ...?

Chapter 16

Inside the ivory tower

I spend most, if not all, of my working day in a brand new, fully integrated, purpose designed, non-PFI building which set back the DoH (and thereby, dear reader - via taxation - you) a cool £60 million. Now, although this may be insufficient an amount to mention in passing to one's cabinet minister spouse over the cornflakes, it nevertheless focuses the mind somewhat. You may well ask in what way the facilities contained within our attractive exterior, justify this sort of expenditure.

Entering via the automatic doors into the two-story high lobby (or atrium) will take your breath away. This is also partly due to the half mile walk from where you eventually managed to park the car, together with the sudden gust of cold air that hits you square in the chops, courtesy of the enormous air conditioning system.

You stroll through wide, brightly lit corridors, past attractive artwork, clip-clopping over mosaic floors, pausing only to admire the marble-effect colonnades. It is then that you start to notice ... the lighting. As you progress along, the ceiling lights ahead of you switch on, and those behind, turn off. Lights that detect movement are not new and presumably save the NHS enormous amounts of cash (yeah, right!). However, they can also lead to bizarre behaviour when assorted staff and patients, suddenly stand tall and dance around waving their arms wildly in an attempt to illuminate a ward thrown abruptly into darkness by an electrical failure.

The computer chip-containing identity card that hangs at a jaunty angle round your neck is carelessly shown to the panel next to each door. There is then a soft 'clunk' as the lock is released, or instead the door itself opens rapidly with a 'ssssshwoop'. I wonder whether the technology used here can actually track the location of the card holder, and thereby - and more importantly - the time actually spent in the building. (It would even be able to differentiate one's presence on the wards or in the labs, from the toilets or coffee room, and thus be in a better position to assess actual time worked). More than once, whilst musing upon the scary possibility of extending this "Big Brother" philosophy, I have been smacked on the hooter by the door which I wrongly assumed was going to open away from me.

The door unlocking/opening system has its own subtleties. A particular entrance to our catheter lab suite has the identity card 'swish' panel placed just too far from the door to allow the entrant to get to there before the system defaults back to 'locked'. It takes a number of vain attempts before you realise that this cannot be accomplished at normal walking pace. You can succeed if the card is flashed whilst sprinting at the portal or, more easily, if an assistant uses his pass behind you. There then follows a Bodie and Doyle (remember them?) type scene as you rush the door. You lean against it to stop it closing while number two runs through. He stops and, SAS-like, checks that you have not been crushed.

You then dive free of the slamming partition, and with the shout "Clear!" you both return calmly from 1970s ITV, to 21st century cardiology.

There are numerous other examples of the degree of thought behind our workplace. An auto valet system allows nursing staff to swish their card in order to get a newly pressed and clean uniform (usually theirs), robotically presented; staff rooms and coffee lounges have boilers supplying instant hot water - not a novel idea, but when you think of the time customarily required to boil a kettle, I suspect a significant saving in man- or more probably, woman-hours.

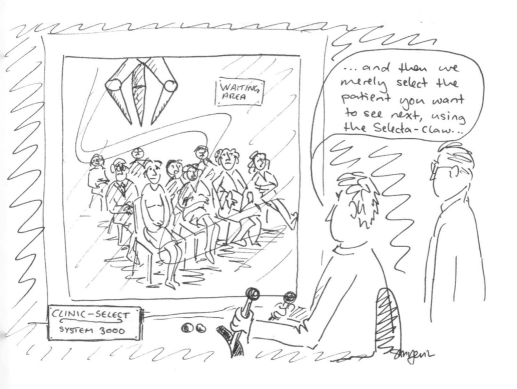

One of the most intriguing technologies is the transportation system that moves blood specimens, prescriptions, messages (and possibly sandwiches) throughout the organisation, driven by compressed air via a complex network of one foot diameter plastic pipes. The ward staff simply load samples into cylindrical 'pods', dial up the destination and wait. Only one pod can travel at a time, presumably to avoid collisions deep in the system; when the line is clear, the specimen is despatched. Nurses are alerted to the imminent arrival of a sample by a rumbling sound in the pipe work, akin to air trapped in a domestic central heating system. The grunting and grinding get louder, until a crescendo is reached, at which point there is an unedifying, but nevertheless satisfying, 'plop'. This accompanies the expulsion into a receiving basket of yet another well travelled pod that has journeyed from the far flung corners of the hospital. Now, tell me that isn't a labour-saving device!

"... suggestions as to other gadgets that might be installed to facilitate the non-clinical functioning of the unit fell upon deaf ears."

Resting ECGs recorded anywhere in the hospital are uploaded wirelessly onto a central server; these together with exercise tests, echoes and angiograms can be viewed on terminals throughout the building. Then there are the security cameras and video entry systems, so that relatives can be vetted before they visit loved ones, and a fire alarm which produces such a brain-dissolving screech that you have to get out of the building as soon as you can if only to escape the din. Then there are the monthly generator tests that result in my office and, crucially, the second floor toilets (neither considered to be an essential clinical area), being suddenly plunged into near darkness, save for dim emergency lighting afforded by nothing more luminescent than a Christmas tree light.

I remain disappointed that the most fundamental device for an interventional cardiologist - and one which would have transformed the working lives of so many of us here - has not materialised; namely, a better way of hanging up protective lead coats. I had envisaged a series of hooks that descend from the ceiling at the swipe of an ID card. They attach to rings at the back of the collar and waist (for the two-piece designs), and gently lift the bloody things from your weary shoulders, thence to be hung way up high, well out the way, safely and - from a chief radiographer's view - correctly.

Sadly, my suggestions as to other gadgets that might be installed to facilitate the non-clinical functioning of the unit fell upon deaf ears. Hence, rather than with bleeps, doctors are frequently summoned on their own mobile phones; this strikes me not only as a tad expensive, but also unreliable if you are stranded and sitting in darkness with poor network coverage (see above). I have always been a fan of tannoy systems such as those that pervade airports and railway stations. They rely on the 'cocktail party theory', i.e. that an individual will be alerted, through low level chit-chat, to his or her own name even if uttered at no more than conversation volume. (I can only presume that from an evolutionary perspective, this innate auditory ability bestowed a survival advantage. Perhaps when Neanderthal man was at a 'bring your own berries' party, it would have been helpful for him to be informed that it was about to be crashed by a hungry sabre-toothed tiger).

There is something reassuring about a continuing background level of monotonous southern-US female drawl that gives a sense of calm efficiency: "Dr. Norell, please pick up a white phone. Dr. Crippin to Gynaecology. Please note: there is an ongoing generator test" (Great!). "There will be a demonstration of manual handling in the first floor seminar room at 1300 hours today. Dr. Norell, please pick up a white phone. Dr. Frankenstein to the mortuary. The fire alarm test originally planned for 0900 will now take place at midday" (Damn!). "There will be a lecture on primary PCI in the 2nd floor library at 1430 hours. Dr. Jekyll, Mr Hyde is waiting for you in main reception. Dr. Norell - white phone, please! ... Security to second floor, washroom six!"

Chapter 17

In the midst of life we are in debt

Perhaps I'm getting old, or maybe have just been in the business for too long (readers would agree with the former as a biological certainty and as for the latter, there are certainly colleagues who might hold that view). However, I do wonder whether contemporaries would recognise my disquiet whilst flicking through the odd broadsheet or occasional tabloid in our coffee room or, whilst brushing teeth, pause and actually listen to the background tones of Radio 5 Live or the Today programme: "NHS Trusts plan redundancies".

Since qualifying in - (skip that bit) - I have tried hard to acquire a working knowledge of our National Health Service. Gradually I appreciated that doctoring was not just about using skills, knowledge and experience as an individual in order to make patients' lives better. As consultants we have to work with our managers in order to be familiar with balancing budgets, revenue, recharging, cost and volume, consumables, commissioning and contracts. Every year we see nervousness around us, as under-, or over-performance looms, and potential 'breachers' come precariously close to targets prompting the stop-start pattern that so often spawns yet another waiting list initiative. (Using the term 'initiative' to describe the apparently novel idea of extra activity, seems to imply a degree of elegance that is unjustified; it is similar to describing the crushing of a coronary side branch stent, by another in the main vessel, as a 'technique').

"As consultants we have to work with our managers in order to be familiar with balancing budgets, revenue, recharging, cost and volume, consumables, commissioning and contracts."

I cannot recollect a time when the many and various financial difficulties of the NHS have ever before led to the contemplation of job losses. We have become depressingly familiar with regrettable announcements of unemployment at Rover, Pilkington's or British Aerospace. We might ponder as to the social consequences, the financial or domestic impact - but not for long. We may breathe a quiet sigh to ourselves: business is business; these things happen. Well, you bet; welcome to the market place!

Decades of under funding, greater healthcare demands and patient expectations, together with an aging population are rolled out limply, albeit as genuine explanations. The use of the NHS as a political football simply aggravates the problem by distracting attention towards short-term (and election-orientated) headlines. This analogy of the 'beautiful game' also applies to the implementation of the recent consultant contract, no doubt to be conveniently cited as the cause of the crisis. It was a major own goal, stemming from the presumption that when senior clinicians actually scrutinised their timetables, the resulting number of Programmed Activities would average out to a convenient ten. Woops!

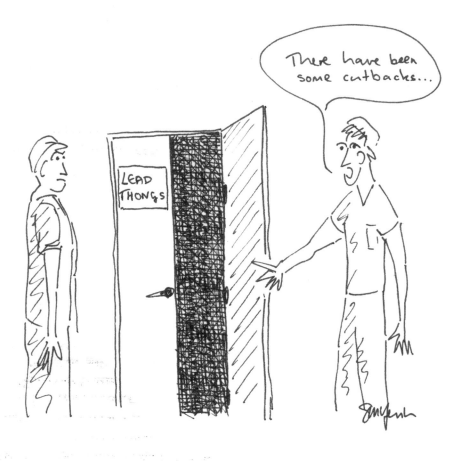

Not so - and thus the last straw fluttered down to nestle between the creaking humps of the NHS camel.

So, as we learn that Trusts are around £800 million in the red, what can be done to balance the books? The NHS has maintained its recognised high level of efficiency by selfless hard work and sacrifice on the part of its staff. Dedication on such a scale is unheard of in the private or commercial sector. If elements of this workforce are now to be dismantled - possibly in the region of many thousands - how will the much heralded future healthcare targets be achieved?

Simply removing sandwiches from lunchtime meetings (the so called 'biscuit budget') is not going to make a huge impact, other than on the odd waistline. (The fact that many of us do not even recognise the phrase 'lunch hour', simply underscores the slightly emotional sentiments - unusual in this book - expressed in the last paragraph). We are currently exploring a mechanical device (better than any human) that provides very effective external cardiac massage. Are we seriously to contemplate that a nursing post on the ward could thus be saved?

There is a philosophy underlying staffing which also applies to enhanced patient flows. Delivering patient care efficiently simply means that the next in line (for there always is one) can be managed more quickly. Similarly, outsourcing dictated letters to Delhi for typing or using computer software to generate reports should not cause a secretary to look forward to receiving her P45. It may allow administrative staff to address other tasks, but you can bet that we will still need them somewhere in the organisation. Such is the truth of a system that is not in balance - with demand always exceeding supply.

An initial response might be to work oneself out of debt by advantageous use of tariffs and the apparently ingenious 'Payment by Results' schemes. However, beware! If you suspect something is too good to be true, it will be. Getting patients with acute coronary syndromes home or returned to their base hospital following an IHT and brisk PCI ('balloon and back'), or repatriated six hours or so after a direct admission for infarct angioplasty ('reperfuse and return'), may seem to be an attractive income generator (let alone, good for patients - I always forget that bit), but one's Trust might not necessarily receive the full tariff whack for such efficiency.

Attempting to devise innovative ways of cashing in on these new arrangements is not rocket science. As far as multi-vessel PCI is concerned, staging patients to form a sequence of single-vessel procedures might keep each one below tariff and thus one's head above the financial water. This is particularly prevalent in some European countries where the financing of healthcare systems encourages such practice. But - best for patients? (There's that word again). I don't think so! One even hears of commissioners declining to cough up for elective activity that is not close to breaching an agreed waiting time target. This perverse contractual loophole means that even if a Trust can keep waiting lists short, and thereby treat patients more quickly, it will not get paid for such efficient work.

It may be a roller coaster ride, but if we focus on what is best for patients we should not go far wrong. The network structures have their foundation on this principle and are further mandated to ensure equity across their respective patches. We still (largely) control who goes on our waiting lists and the much trumpeted targets will then automatically demand timely treatment. We cannot decline urgent cases; emerging acceptable inter-hospital transfer times should again work in the patients' favour - always assuming that we aspire to a meaningful standard of, say, 48 hours rather than a more 'achievable' delay (for some unearthly reason) of two weeks.

In the last few years the NHS has been the happy recipient of significant and unparalleled financial attention and cardiology particularly, has seen tangible improvements as a result. The honeymoon is now over; belts will soon need to be tightened again. We stand a better prospect of getting through the years ahead if we work as genuine teams, both in our departments and across our networks. In the meantime we can take reassurance in the notion that potential job losses may occur as a result of 'natural wastage'. Well - that's the polite way of putting it!

Chapter 18

The angioplasty apprentice

Previously I have made comments on the subject of cardiological teaching - history taking, murmurs, etc. (*Cardiology News passim*) - but I wish to focus this contribution upon the more specific area of interventional training.

My colleagues and I work in a semi-surgical specialty. I say this not because we employ a heavy duty anaesthetic, or make huge incisions releasing large amounts of blood (hang on a minute ...), but because we use manual skills to realise a defined clinical endpoint, the quality of which is directly related to our expertise. This marks us out from other physicians; a patient's response to a thoughtfully prescribed drug is not directly attributable to their handiwork.

As a result, we find ourselves in a similar position to our surgical colleagues when educating, monitoring and supervising, before eventually signing off our trainees. What processes need to be employed to ensure that we can be as confident as possible that our dedicated protégés can be unleashed safely onto a trusting public?

We begin with suitable material; individuals selected increasingly by interview during the latter half of their formal training programme, are slotted into registrar posts specifically formatted to supply concentrated and structured interventional exposure in their final two years. They will have a sound foundation in cardiac catheterisation and will have shown themselves to be 'hands positive'.

This is a tricky quality to assess objectively. It is not enough just to watch in order to make a judgement; I yell from the back of the lab as a right Judkins catheter gyrates randomly around the ascending aorta, making occasional forays into the left ventricle. "Stop. Start again higher up. LAO. Point towards 3 o'clock, slowly turn clockwise and watch it drop ... no more than 180 degrees." Sometimes they look puzzled when I suggest that they torque too much.

I know that the substrate is good when I sense my mind controlling their actions, i.e. 'your head in their hands'. Just pulling on a pair of gloves (after washing, of course), and a lead coat (perhaps not in that order), before engaging the right coronary artery yourself, is hardly doing your trainee any favours. You could always mess it up, deliberately taking another ten minutes to succeed in order to rebuild their confidence. They need to demonstrate a reaction to what they see. "Move, then test. Move, then test", therefore rings out frequently above the background melodies of Dean Martin.

Training styles undoubtedly differ. Operators - like drivers - tend to feel that the only correct way of doing it is their way. However, angioplasty has become increasingly forgiving; although there are definite 'no-nos', there are nevertheless many right ways to skin the interventional cat, so to speak. Trainees would benefit from selecting samples from a range of teachers, if possible. I was mentored according to the 'teaching by confrontation' philosophy. My own style has lapsed into more of a Gordon Ramsey technique, which can be a problem depending on the acoustics in the lab, our trainee's sensitivities and the patient's hearing.

How do we define the role of trainees in each case, particularly in terms of first or second operator? Surely it is not simply a question of who stands where - 'front-ending', as it is rather unfortunately termed. Decision-making is the dominant skill, with manual dexterity a clear second. Although patients are ultimately the responsibility of the consultant trainer, we can still allow the case to be executed (sorry, conducted) by our fellows, and thereby bestow the title of primary operator upon them retrospectively after the case debriefing.

"The thought processes involved are crucial; thinking perhaps three or more steps ahead, anticipating all likely eventualities from any action and always having an alternative strategy."

There is this obsession with numbers. If we were to believe all our trainees, their own interventional volumes would exceed the annual total derived from all UK units. Certainly, and paradoxically, the more you do the more interesting each case becomes. Similarly the golfing analogy, "the more you practice, the luckier you get", holds true in the catheter lab just as on the first tee at Turnbury (writing as one whose umpteenth drive once concussed a sheep).

The thought processes involved are crucial; thinking perhaps three or more steps ahead, anticipating all likely eventualities from any action and always having an alternative strategy. There is a similarity with sailing here: knowing where the nearest safe port might be in case of a storm, or as with the SAS apparently, having an escape route planned if things go 'noisy' (sic). The often-used Norellism is, "if you don't know what you're going to do next, you shouldn't be doing what you're doing now".

What else can help? Meetings and live courses are always worthwhile. The occasional pinch of salt should be available in order to provide the necessary reality check when a first-year registrar from another centre describes his personal experience of stenting 54 consecutive quadrification lesions. Books? Well, only one springs to mind, namely *Essential Interventional Cardiology*; editors Norell & Perrins, publishers Harcourt and available from Amazon at £39.95 - apparently. (That's enough of that! Ed.).

Eventually, after demoting oneself to second operator, and then withdrawing to the back of the lab, the coffee room and finally one's office, we have to cut the umbilical and let our young guns fly solo. While the patients remain under our care, trainees must nevertheless make their own mistakes and then get out of the problem themselves. It is now that the trainer appreciates the value of previously not rushing in so soon in order to help out. Indeed, after eventually showing our fellow how to wire a particularly tricky vessel, I have been known to purposefully remove the wire in order to get him to do it himself!

When the apprenticeship is over, the product of our training can take his or her place as a stand-alone operator. They may now work independently but that is not to imply that they function in isolation. Increasingly, senior colleagues work in teams, sharing experiences and providing mutual support. This is particularly important - and should be assumed - when our protégés embark on their own consultant career.

Perhaps, when they are in the middle of a tricky case they will hear a loud voice with an East End London accent from the back of the lab, which will remind them of their years spent training and give them renewed confidence to complete the case: "That guiding catheter is the wrong shape and should be 7 French; both wires must be supportive with more tip angulation for the marginal branch; you should have predilated the main vessel with a shorter balloon; that stent is too long and you should have used Reopro. You're fired!"

Chapter 19

It's not what you say, but how you say it

I step warily into this particular subject area, anxious not to irritate, upset or annoy those whose use of the English Language derives from anywhere other than BBC Radio 4. Even this bastion of correctness has been gradually infiltrated by a welcome array of contributions from our home nations. Thus, helpful magazine programmes centering on health issues, and particularly female maladies, are introduced by warm Welsh tones direct from the Rhonda. Reviews and analyses of recent political intrigues are accompanied by a soft Edinburgh brogue, whilst probing and provocative exposés about unscrupulous builders defrauding an octogenarian widow are headed up by a harsh Belfast twang.

Is there intelligent design behind such planning? I am sure the answer is yes, and now wish to extend this observation into more familiar territory. Could some fundamental cardiological elements, with which we are familiar in day to day practice, be subconsciously linked to different accents? I have alluded previously to the Lieutenant Colombo approach to history taking (Added Sounds, *passim*), but to what extent might Jacques Cousteau assist in the physical examination of the heart?

"We descend further, the diaphragm of our simple stethoscope gliding gently over the praecordium. We are greeted by a soft, pansystolic whoosh that becomes increasingly audible, its rhythmic tones jostling playfully in our ears, as if to bid us welcome to the enchanted and mysterious world of mitral regurgitation."

ECG and arrhythmia analysis will always be - in my view at least - the area in which our own countrymen excel. The degree of preciseness required to describe an apparently chaotic cardiac rhythm, or the multi-channel recordings spewed out after a four-hour-long accessory pathway ablation, demands the cool, clipped, Saville Row sharpness of an English electrophysiologist.

> "Could some fundamental cardiological elements, with which we are familiar in day to day practice, be subconsciously linked to different accents?"

As for heart failure, well, think about it. Of all the presentations you have witnessed, which one accent seems to encapsulate the care and consideration required to deal with this huge long-term health problem, as well as the authority and confidence to interpret and react rapidly to the results of multimillion dollar drug trials? Quite right! Anything close to Sean Connery will do here as this is undoubtedly the domain of our northern neighbours. I am certain that in order to get a consultant appointment with a special interest in left ventricular dysfunction, you have to conduct your interview like Billy Connolly - at least in terms of accent. Shut you eyes and hear yourself saying the following in the guise of one of our many colleagues north of Hadrian's Wall: "Haaart Faylyerrrh!" Now, am I right or am I right?

What of cardiological trials generally? Which nation seems to have an unenviable grasp of the data and the objectivity to broadcast it in an acceptable form? I would suggest the Scandinavians. They gave us beta-blockers after AMI, ACE inhibitors in CHF, statins in CHD and Danami in Primary PCI. We cannot but take them seriously. Their accent on the other hand requires a certain degree of tolerance; there is a painstaking pace at which their message comes across, perhaps exemplified by the following dialogue, overheard in a Danish chemist's shop, and which needs to be read at one third normal speed:

Customer: "I would like to buy a deodorant please".

Shopkeeper: "Certainly. Ball or aerosol?"

Customer: "Neither. It's for my armpit".

PCI has given new impetus to some of these accents. Many of us cut our teeth at courses organised by Geoff Hartzler and colleagues at the Mid-America Heart Institute in Kansas City, Missouri. The drawl with which he described a very acceptable angiographic result as "none too shabby" is still used by many of us today. The US influence is still prevalent, with the TCT meetings in Washington being a major global event. None of the many dialects to be heard there are particularly memorable; they all blend into one smooth North American generic, announcing and greeting each faculty member as their "closest and dearest friend".

That is not to deny that the Dutch and French accents have a major influence here. The former pioneered coronary stenting courses at the

OLGV and Erasmus University hospitals, particularly from the radial arterial approach. The cadence of their language has a particular resonance and familiarity with our own tongue. The latter led the way in Toulouse and Paris and must have influenced many thousands of operators across the world, not only with their techniques but also in the way they used certain terms that are commonplace in interventional practice. I cannot be the only one who, on returning from such a meeting, find myself lapsing into similar, Clouseau-like pronunciations of words like 'millimetres' (millimeerrrt) or 'manoeuvre' (mannerve).

Certain interventional techniques or devices can only be employed with an Italian accent. We cannot treat a bifurcation lesion with crush stenting successfully unless we talk to ourselves as we do it: "Eet iza vary importanta to ensure zatta the proximale enda ova the sida brancha stenta iza covered bya the proximale enda ova the stenta een the main vessele."

And what of cardiac rehabilitation; how do we incorporate this NSF chapter, and essential part of the care package, into our international language template? Is there a national stereotype which encapsulates almost military efficiency, strict regimentation, regular exercise and dietary routines, self discipline and camaraderie - all part and parcel of a rehab programme? Let me have a think while I take this beach towel off the treadmill.

Chapter 20

Ten atmospheres and all that

I'd rather assumed that most readers would be familiar with all the various words and terms related to PCI, which are bandied about by me every month or so in the columns of the *British Journal of Cardiology* and *Cardiology News*. However - possibly not. So, in an attempt to correct this oversight on my part, I am pleased to submit the following as a 'beginner's guide' to coronary intervention.

Result, final (angiographic): the eventual outcome of the procedure, usually - but not always - documented by the last X-ray acquisition.

Good result: undoubtedly better than before.

Acceptable result: not quite 'good' (see above), but the operator cannot think of anything else that might improve things further.

Excellent result: perfect and indistinguishable from a normal artery. (Technical point: this term only applies when the artery was abnormal before the procedure).

First operator: 1. Named individual who is going to have a first crack at the case (not necessarily the most senior team member). 2. The guy who (decided after completion of the procedure) has been selected to take the flack if things go belly-up (certainly not the most senior team member).

"...a 'beginner's guide' to coronary intervention."

Second operator: 1. Usually an assistant (nurse or trainee) whose job it is to stop the first operator from dropping expensive pieces of kit on the lab floor. 2. The guy who steps in after the first operator has messed things up, big-time.

High pressure: sense of anxiety felt by first operator trainees.

Pressure wire: 1. Hurriedly attempting to cross with a guide wire a complex, critically stenosed or subtotally occluded last remaining vessel, when your outpatient clinic started ten minutes ago. 2. Relatively expensive device used to confirm that you did the right thing not to stent that lesion which looked no more than 30% on angiography. (See also: 'Mark-1 Eyeball').

Torque: 1. Property of a catheter or wire allowing rotation at the proximal end to produce a similar and predictable deflection at the distal tip. Excessive torque is undesirable, and can distract the operator who will then ask to keep the bloody noise down. 2. The resulting improvement following a quiet word with a trainee who is underperforming (as in, '1:1 torque response').

O-Ring: 1. Device attached to guide catheter allowing to and fro movement of wires, balloons etc, without undue back-bleeding or loss of pressure monitoring. (See also: haemostatic valve, haemoglobin and transfusion). 2. Eventual, sighing agreement by trainee after lab staff have pleaded with him for two hours to phone his consultant for help.

Y-Connector: curious but essential implement, incorporating O-Ring (see above), used to test assistants' familiarity with interventional equipment. (The question, "why?", is predictably followed by them connecting it back to front).

OTW: Over The Wire. Early balloon catheter design - still in use today - with guide wire passing through whole length of shaft. See also: 1. Excessive high pressure expansion or unnecessary multiple stents in already perfectly treated lesion (OTT, Over The Top). 2. Procedure undertaken by trainee with advice from consultant still in his office (OTP, Over The Phone).

Monorail: ingeniously simple - and patented - balloon catheter design that you wish you had thought of first. (See also: rapid exchange; taking cath lab blues off and dressing quickly in order to get to private clinic).

DES: 1. Drug-eluting stent. Expensive, but worthwhile technological advance, produced by dipping a BMS (Bare Metal Stent) in goats' entrails and holy water. 2. Frequent request for background music in cath lab, as in "Give me some Frank, Dean, Nat or Des".

Low profile: used to describe operator who is virtually unheard of. (Opposite of: high profile; an operator who is anywhere but working in his own unit).

IVUS: Intra-Vascular UltraSound. Infrequently used but nevertheless valuable diagnostic device that can differentiate intravascular anatomy and tissue types. As in: calcified (white), non-calcified (black), fatty-fibrous (black and white), fibro-fatty (white and black), crescentric calcification (black with white line), intimal disruption or dissection (white with black line), thrombus (sort of greyish, or straight line; see also: ECG). Opposite in function to pressure wire, i.e. its use is *more* likely to provoke intervention.

Kiss: 1. Simultaneous inflation of adjacent balloons or stents, used particularly in bifurcation lesions. 2. Paradoxically, acronym for "Keep It Simple, Stupid", warning operators NOT to make cases unnecessarily complicated.

Crush: 1. Elegant technique used to treat bifurcation lesions. (See also: Culottes, Provisional T, V, Y and 'pain in the backside'). 2. Restricted cath lab changing facilities.

Bifurcation lesion: stenosis situated proximal, distal or at, a branch point (i.e. nearly all cases). These have been angiographically classified A-G, depending on where plaque is evident. Trifurcation lesions have been classified A-O, confirming that - in PCI at any rate - there are some really sad anoraks that should get out more.

Over-inflation: applied to operator's CV; relates to number of personal first operator cases alleged to have been performed, which exceeds the unit's total.

Strategy: plan cobbled together after the case in the hope of giving colleagues the impression that you knew what you were doing at the beginning. Also used, as figure of speech: "I elected to ...", meaning, "At this point I got desperate".

In-deflator: used during a long and exhausting case; an early sign of operator confusion.

CTO: Chronic Total Occlusion. A lesion with a predictable low success rate, and therefore a description applied retrospectively - after operator has failed to stent it. (Alternative meaning: Couldn't Treat Optimally).

Success: originally defined as achievement of <50% stenosis, with no clinical complication. Although still used by some, term now modified to take account of vastly improved outcomes with stenting. Also: complete success (as in, "All done, bish-bash-bosh"), and partial success (as in, "He was OK until he got back to the ward").

Canute: (Orig. King Canute, 994-1035. English monarch famed for attempting to halt the incoming tide). Derogatory term applied to colleague who is reluctant to take on new and proven technologies; as in, "He's a bit of a Canute". (Care with spelling required).

POBA: Plain Old Balloon Angioplasty. Quaint and romantic term, harking back to a bygone era, and applied to treatment using balloon dilatation alone, and no stent. A major resurgence in use is anticipated as a result of NHS funding cuts.

Protected left main: high risk and complex lesion subset, only to be undertaken after surgeons have given you the "OK", and you have cleared it with the MDU. (See also: 'No surgical back-up'; used when the surgeon denies any discussions with him beforehand).

No reflow: peculiar phenomenon in which the quality of the final result (see above) is inversely related to the extent of treatment. (See also: O-Ring, MDU and 'Reasons for late religious conversion').

UKCCAD: rather old fashioned, accusatory expression used when an operator realises a colleague has fiddled his own PCI audit returns in order to make himself look good. (See also: 'You lying bas***d!').

Chapter 21

Our mission: to boldly state ...

Most people don't notice them. Or perhaps just glance. Some might take no more than a passing interest as they scan a letterhead, footer or billboard. Others have no choice but to observe the back of the van they are stuck behind or the side of the truck as they are eventually able to overtake. What phenomenon is this? I suppose it is best summed up as 'the philosophy'; a few words painstakingly combined over many hours, which succinctly describe an organisation's raison d'être. Its motivation or organisational ethos, its mission or positioning statement.

Apparently, if more than one person is employed, then no self respecting firm, society, business or multimillion dollar, multinational conglomerate, can hold up its head in the market place without one. Why is this? From where did these phrases come and what purpose do they serve? What demarcates a memorable and witty use of a few choice words, as opposed to 21st century business-like twaddle and a complete waste of some focus group's energy, time and money?

"These **phrases** need to **work** on a **number** of **levels**. They need to be **grammatically correct** for a start. They need to **express** what the **organisation** is quintessentially **about**..."

I found myself engaged in this quest when involved in a video conference call earlier this year. Instead of spending five hours down and up the M40 in a vain attempt to attend a two-hour meeting, I suggested utilising some modern gadgetry instead. It meant that I missed out on some impressively novel sandwiches, as well as the opportunity to finish one or two articles on my laptop whilst sitting between J10 and J11 (*Br J Cardiol, passim*), but the time saved was just about worth it. In order to link up, I had to get onto the website of the firm that hosted such contact, and it was there that I was struck by their understated strap line: "We must start meeting like this." Now, is that clever or is that clever?

These phrases need to work on a number of levels. They need to be grammatically correct for a start. They need to express what the organisation is quintessentially about, and frequently incorporate double - or even treble - entendres that allow the casual (or in some cases the more often anally-retentive) reader to appreciate all the underlying, subliminal and interspersed messages contained therein. The most common seem to incorporate the words 'logistics' or 'solutions'. In the latter case the only company I could think of that might successfully utilise that element would be a fully staffed Israeli or Jordanian business specialising in the export of surplus sodium chloride from the Dead Sea ('Saturated Salt Solutions').

The relevance to cardiological matters is two-fold. Many pharmaceutical and device companies have incorporated these catchphrases, and may consider them as some form of mantra - perhaps seen in the mind's eye as surrounded by a Turner-esque sunset, steaming rain forest, calm ocean or snow covered mountain peak,

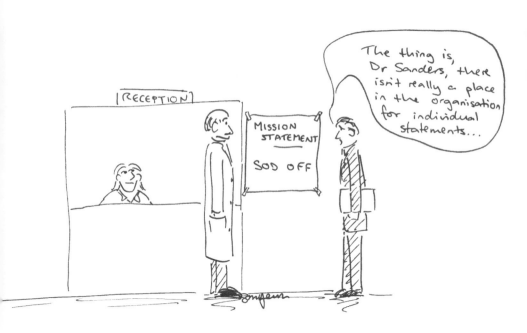

which their representatives have to visualise as they promote their organisation. "Delivering what's next", is a current example from a forward thinking device business, although to me it seems more suited to a busy midwife. Interestingly, in this particular case, the phrase has been copyrighted (or patented), so that's bad luck for the Post Office as well.

I have tried without success to legally protect, in a similar way, a phrase of my own: the "Triangle of Death" aptly describes the anatomy and consequences of inadequate stent coverage of a side branch ostium when addressing a bifurcation lesion. (I can't imagine why the general public are not the least bit interested in this; every four years our nation's football team find themselves qualifying for the World Cup in the "Group of Death". This predictable description is designed to anticipate a stormy course and thereby justify in advance our early departure from the competition). As for branch vessel angioplasty, my silk has had no luck thus far, but I would still warn you to use this phrase at your peril.

The second reason relates to the British Cardiac (sorry, Cardiovascular) Society and its ongoing re-branding exercise. I could not discern any parallel message or secondary meaning in "Promoting Cardiovascular Health". It is simple enough, easy to understand and non-provocative; understated, unambiguous and undeniable. (Who said unnecessary?)

The more we become aware of this trend, the more of these we will notice. Just last week I saw "Health and safety is no accident" on a placard adorning a building site, and on a water company compressor attending to a minor sewerage problem (wait for it ...), "Your waste safe in our hands" (... and I kid you not!).

Examples of poorly produced statements are numerous, although sometimes they deliberately appear clumsy in order to increase the likelihood that you will remember the particular business or product. I have no doubt that the florists who boldly announced: "If your mother-in-law is at death's door, our flowers will pull her through", saw their stock rise considerably.

Ethereal and futuristic sentences suggest that the company in question has "seen the light" and that it is only a matter of time before everyone else catches up with their unique working practice. Hence, "Someday, all banks/garages/taxidermists will be run this way", gives a warm sense of confidence as we leave our money, car or much-loved household pet in their charge.

There remains one classic line that enshrined succinctly the ultimate corporate philosophy, capturing perfectly the essence and ethos of the organisation. The fact that the English speaking public found "Vorschsprung durch technik" completely unintelligible, simply enhanced its strength, mystery and vision, and thereby its authority and the confidence it engendered. Sheer genius!

Chapter 22

The conference bag

To start with, I am not referring here to the regular political get-togethers that punctuate the autumn or spring seasons in Brighton or Harrogate; happily this is not about Anne Widecombe or Claire Short.

I found myself clearing out a garage recently and it was while knee deep in back copies of Yachting Monthly, expired passports (you would not believe the photographs) and broken lamps, I came across a hoard of them. Cowering in a dark corner, together as if for protection; there they all were. Spiders' webs, damp-rot and mill dew had tarnished them understandably, but slapping them against a brick wall and avoiding the resulting cloud of dust, soon restored their original significance: Cardiostim, Monte Carlo, 1985; Acute PTCA, Geneva, 1986; Fifth World Congress on Primary Care, Manila, 1972 (a classic, and one of my father's, presumably).

A major conference or meeting nowadays is not complete without attendees collecting a recognisable trophy of their experience in the form of a case, haversack or recyclable string bag proclaiming the nature, venue and timing of the particular event. What are the origins of this tradition? Is there still a purpose for such large-scale provision of these accessories? Could there be a rain forest, rubber plantation or even small, brown-eyed, furry animal somewhere, that is either being denuded or hunted to extinction, in an attempt to feed the insatiable desire for these needless items?

I can only presume that they were originally supplied to answer a particular need. The pharmaceutical and the device industries support international conferences with astonishingly sophisticated exhibitions and phenomenally well stocked stands (as well as delegates' registration, accommodation and travel expenses). The result is an increasingly bizarre selection of give-away items such as pens, clocks, reading lamps, mints, lollipops, umbrellas, hats, paperweights and, not to mention, squeezy, soft, rubbery stress relieving balls (they don't work, by the way). Somehow these valued objects have to be transported around the congress centre, and then back home to your loved ones to be presented as a hard thought-about coming home present, in something a tad larger than your jacket pocket.

"Is there still a purpose for such large-scale provision of these accessories?"

Then there is the 'course material': the final programme, abstract book, exhibitors' catalogue, a collection of spurious reprints from various journals pertinent to the meeting, invitations to numerous evening satellite meetings at which refreshments and canapés (but not din-dins) are available and a map of the city just in case you did not know where the congress was this year. There are the 'factoids': a small - but substantial - tome, summarising succinctly every trial conducted that is in any way relevant to the conference theme; the pen - conveniently with a torch combined - so that you, and everyone else, can make frantic notes in the darkness of the main auditorium and thereby give the speaker the sense that his session has been invaded by a swarm of fireflies; the mouse pad adorned with the conference logo and website; cath lab scrub suits, jogging vests, track suit tops and 'sweat' pants (I think that's what they're called).

Crucially there is also the personal, embossed invitation to the Gala night. This is usually arranged for the penultimate night of the congress, now clashing with your recently - and hastily - arranged flight home. It may be at the local museum, opera house or bull ring and features abundant food and drink (thank goodness for that!), street theatre, magic shows, fireworks and some demonstration of the national culture such as caber-tossing, Morris or clog dancing or bell ringing. (I remember one such event in Geneva featuring a re-enactment of William Tell -

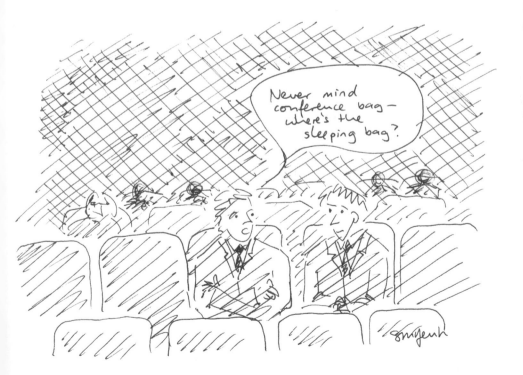

including son and apple - together with an impersonator who, for every subject, pushed his dinner jacket back over his shoulders, squinted, blew out his cheeks and looked like Popeye. This seemed to work for Popeye but for no-one else - at least that the UK contingent could recognise).

The most useful inclusions I seem to remember were as part of a course in Paris, and comprised a collection of Metro tickets, while the bag adorned with "2nd Annual Conference on Cytochrome P450 and its Modulation in Systemic Disease, Helsinki" did not immediately make me feel that this was a meeting I just *had* to be at. The fact that the bags are identical adds to the uniformity and esprit de coeur that the conference might hope to generate in its attendees, but it adds also a degree of confusion in the queue for security X-ray scanning at the airport on the way home.

A PCI course in Toulouse a decade or so ago, provided a T-shirt on the back of which were (in a fairly small font) the names of all the delegates (I eventually found mine - spelled incorrectly as usual). They also produced a hard-backed 'course curriculum' that must have been at least four inches thick. Luckily, they also provided a fairly stalwart rucksack for the purpose of lugging all this stuff home (but which I still use).

The modern era has seen computer bags replace the more attaché case-looking items. I - and my kids - have certainly found them useful but whether I need to get a new one at each conference is debatable. They seem to have far more pockets than I need; I recognise the one for a mobile phone (presumably) but I struggle to work out what I am supposed to slip into the others. Course organisers realise that most of us bring our laptops to conferences, and the sad thing is that they are probably right. Huge and unwieldy volumes of course materials have been replaced with a slim CD on which one can find the programme, abstracts, presentations and - if you're really lucky - the Popeye impersonator.

Chapter 23

"We are, where we are"

The above title struck me as wholly appropriate for this chapter. The only problem was going to be how I could weave in, almost imperceptibly, any conceivable cardiological relevance. Well, here goes ...

Like it or not, 21st century cardiology is a fast lane specialty. The clinical conditions with which our patients present require our immediate attention, whilst even our non-clinical commitments demand our urgent and undivided involvement as departmental budgets of perhaps millions of pounds plus are discussed. So how can we ensure that as little time as possible is spent driving from one unit to another, to a workshop in one of yet another identical hotel chains (see *The Oblique View, passim*) or to the local PCT or ambulance trust - often out of region, and therefore away from familiar territory? How do we avoid getting lost in a faceless industrial estate or, as I have done once when late for an unusually vital meeting, coming to a screeching halt in the middle of a cemetery (and a funeral service in full 'swing'). The answer: in-car satellite navigation. Now, how is that for imperceptible weaving?

Having a hankering after all things nautical, I had got a hand-held device some years ago and used it on my yacht. Undoubtedly useful, it revealed not only latitude and longitude, but also my altitude. The idea that I should be anywhere other than at sea level was a little disconcerting. Science has moved on; the American military, which originally controlled the satellite technology, has allowed even more accurate positioning to be readily accessible to a truly global audience. So now, my boat lights up as a flashing icon zigzagging off Harwich, and an individual's position anywhere on the surface of the planet can be immediately available.

> "How could such an innocent piece of software be anything other than a positive boon to the cardiologist of today?"

Do we really need it in our cars? Well, I thought not, but then was advised by a colleague to make a mental note of just how often such assistance would have truly helped. It did not take long. All you need is a 9.00 a.m. IHT/ACS process-mapping exercise at some forgettable hotel in Leamington Spa, a jack-knifed lorry on the M42 and a comprehensive A-Z of the West Midlands. The final touch is forgetting to bring your reading glasses; the result: incandescence - and the unscheduled gate crashing of an internment (see above).

The current array of systems, whether factory fitted or portable, are all fairly similar. Up to a dozen or more satellites pick up your signal and using triangulation (a process originally invented by the Swiss in order to manufacture Toblerone), overly your position on preinstalled road maps.

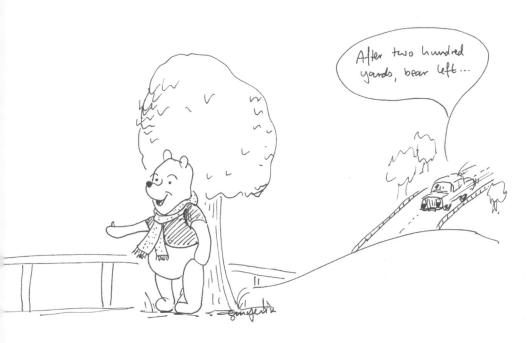

Pop in the post code, house number, road name, or nearest fish and chip shop, on the touch sensitive screen, and it will compute the quickest route for you. If you want to avoid the road works on the M5 (they're still there, by the way), the centre of Worcester or your mother-in-law, it will do all that as well, and then display your ideal route. By monitoring your speed, it will give you a constantly updated ETA and provide a series of instructions and turning prompts, timed perfectly according to how rapidly you are approaching the next junction.

There is a real sense of satisfaction when, as you drive into the vast guest parking area of the Holiday Inn, you hear, "You have arrived at your destination"; a victory of man - in partnership with science - over nature, and all the road works, one way streets and traffic cones she can throw at you. How could such an innocent piece of software be anything other than a positive boon to the cardiologist of today? Well ...

Firstly there's the voice. Yes, you can select from a large range of sex (two there, obviously), ethnic origins and vocal types. I have a preference for 'Jane', a softly spoken lady from Kent - or thereabouts - who, in a refined aircraft cabin attendant sort of way, quietly suggests, "Turn around where possible", when I have ignored instructions or inadvertently missed an exit. Presumably this software is a preinstalled and more polite alternative to, "Are you deaf or something, you bald git?"(I am sorely tempted to keep taking the wrong turns just to see whether the device eventually gives up and defaults to the more basic feminine response of "OK, stop the car. I'm walking!").

Or you could choose an American twang to give the impression that you are somewhere in orbit around the moon, taking instructions from Mission Control in Houston, rather than on the North Circular Road: "We have you one mile from rendezvous at this time. Mark. Please prepare for M-way egress at Junction 14; that is J for Juliet oner-fower."

I get slightly concerned when travelling on a newly constructed road which is not yet part of the system's recognised series of preinstalled maps. Whereas I know that I am on the new bit of the A1(M) or the M6 Toll, my Sat-Nav thinks I am either going the wrong way up the River Ouse or ploughing through an enormous turnip field. Its repetitive and futile attempts to update and replan my route could result in a catastrophic shutdown. Dalek-like wails of "Cannot compute! Cannot compute!", would be followed by a minor explosion, littering bits of its innards (wire, plastic and presumably gunky, mushy, brain stuff), all over my dash board and the inside of my windscreen.

There is a more sinister aspect to all this; the idea that - using modern mobile phone technology - someone, somewhere can know exactly where you are anywhere in the world (or hospital, for that matter), and with refined CCTV and security systems, can also get a handle on what you are up to. They could, for instance, even tell when you were in the cath lab, coffee room, office or even - God forbid! - the outpatient clinic. As long as you keep to the speed limit, always park legally and never try to zip across on amber, then the spy in the sky should leave you well alone. But, should you err and come off the A453 too early into a turnip field, then woe betide you!

Chapter 24

Signs

Working within any organisation one becomes accustomed to an environment which, to an outsider, must feel decidedly alien. Every attempt is made to allow the public image to be as open and comprehensible as possible, in the same way as with the customer accessible areas of police stations (of which I have no specific knowledge, by the way) or airports. But as far as hospital-based workers are concerned, it is only when we end up on the receiving end of 'Health Care Delivery' that we are obliged to see ourselves as others see us.

A slightly late re-entry into fatherhood caused me to muse on this notion recently and, finding myself attending an antenatal clinic, I just looked around and got to thinking ...

Firstly there is the basic external sign-posting. This starts at the main road entrance and guides us to those departments which the public are most likely to require: the laundry, chiropody and the mortuary. Directions to the 'Pay and Display' parking areas are supplemented by illuminated - and randomly generated - figures supposedly indicating the number of available free spaces. These turn out to be reasonably accurate just so long as you are prepared to park up on a flowerbed, fence or one-foot-high curb, thereby realising the true purpose of your off-road gas-guzzler.

Then there is the basic geographical layout of the organisation; just as with airports or hotels, hospitals are constructed according to a standard formula. Whether in Schipol or the lobby of the Meridien in Paris, one knows instinctively where the toilets are likely to be, even without the help of the silhouetted couple which has become the iconic and internationally recognised sign for the loo. Similarly, in a patient waiting area, you just know where you are likely to find the flower stall, newsagent or cash machine, all (particularly the last) vital resources for the expectant father.

I recall working in one hospital where the internal routes to the A & E department, pathology or main X-ray were marked by different coloured footprints (with smaller ones heading to the paediatric ward). You would stride diligently along endless corridors, head-down as you religiously followed your assigned pathway, hardly noticing others who were doing the same thing. Collisions and polite apologies were therefore commonplace. The painted shoe patterns even led into the changing cubicles and onto the X-ray table itself; one might have almost expected to see miniature footprints appearing across the subsequently developed X-ray film.

Whether loitering in the waiting area or passing time just by wandering aimlessly along ward corridors, the extraordinary array of notices, posters and announcements make their real impact. We are bombarded by a blunderbuss of messages, each conveniently encompassed in A3 or A4 format. Flyers giving advanced notice of 'upcoming' conferences lie side by side with advertisements for mandatory training sessions and tables converting kilogrammes to their equivalent in stones and pounds. I would suggest that the latter is best avoided, particularly if sited close to a digital weighing machine and next to the green, yellow, orange and red nomogram that plots your weight against your height and thus indicates proudly whether you are pleasingly svelte or a lard-arse.

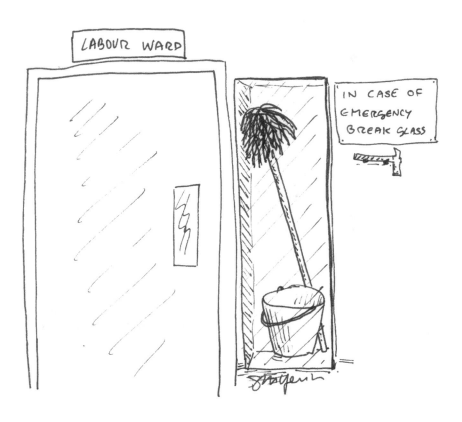

It is simply human nature: there are the scales and you have all the time in the world on your hands. You automatically step on and after a few seconds the red LED display stabilises. You stare aghast, alternating your gaze between the electronic readout and your position on the aforementioned 'Chart of Death' which has been helpfully positioned at face height in front of you. You think to yourself, "I really do not need to know this right now", as you rapidly calculate just how much your shoes, clothes, watch, mobile phone and loose change, might actually weigh in order to bring you into the 'safe zone' and thereby increase the chances of you still being around when your new infant has her first birthday.

"To us, who pass by these images day in day out, they appear second nature and barely impinge on our consciousness. But I do wonder what our patients and their families make of this ..."

A colourful cartoon demonstrating graphically that "we are what we eat" is blue-tacked next to a photograph of a dissected cigarette exposing its porridge-like innards and thereby reminding us that smoking might not exactly be a sensible thing to do. And nestling amongst glossy posters of the department's submissions to various scientific meetings, is - naturally - the ward's mission statement or its "philosophy of care".

This sits nicely alongside the announcement that abusive language or violent behaviour towards hospital staff will not be tolerated - or else! (Huzzah! ... or else what, exactly?).

A relatively recent addition to the abundant literature that adorns the otherwise dull and faded magnolia walls are the innovative and varied reminders of the importance of personal hygiene and disinfection, both contributing to the armamentarium in the newly waged battle against MRSA. One has to acknowledge that these posters are eye catching and clever, if not slightly amusing, but whether they will produce the desired result remains to be seen.

Just as our cardiology wards have the ubiquitous Frank Netter illustrations of cross-sectioned ventricles and graphic displays of coronary arteries, atheroma, stents and balloons, maternity units are similarly festooned. The overwhelming advantages of breast feeding are amply described, such as encouragement of maternal bonding and enhanced infant immunity. Mothers, who are keen to relate to their new born as early as possible, are prompted to discuss with their midwife the possibility of an immediate "skin on skin, contact experience" with their recent arrival. A phone number to use if one is contemplating a birthing pool sits alongside another offering support for would-be mothers at risk of domestic violence.

To us, who pass by these images day in day out, they appear second nature and barely impinge on our consciousness. But I do wonder what our patients and their families make of this mass of clinical or administrative information. Perhaps just one less cigarette or sausage roll, one pair of cleaner hands and a little more politeness, will make it all worth while ... at least until you try to peel off the "Your vehicle is parked in an inappropriate location!" notice from your front windscreen.

Chapter 25

Now wash your hands

Aseptic technique has never been my strong point. I suspect that this is quite fortuitous as infection related to PCI is almost unheard of. (Getting scientific for just a moment, I acknowledge that puncture site sepsis is a well recognised - if uncommon - complication, but this is invariably the result of inadequate haemostasis in the first place, with haematoma or false aneurysm formation subsequently getting infected by groin dwelling bugs. Enough of science, then).

Very occasionally the back end of a guide wire may brush against an injudiciously positioned drip stand. The operator is then faced with two choices: he can sigh and instruct his assistant not to touch anything as he carefully removes the wire (which required forty-five minutes to cross the target lesion) and then starts all over again; or, he can do what I - and some of you - do, namely wipe the end of the wire with a damp swab, and with the reassuring commentary, "Play on, says the referee", go ahead and stent the thing.

The Department of Health's declared crusade against MRSA has unleashed a number of new initiatives. One of these is the idea that reminding caring professionals how to wash their hands prior to undertaking aseptic procedures, will go some way at least to slow the advance of this undesirable organism.

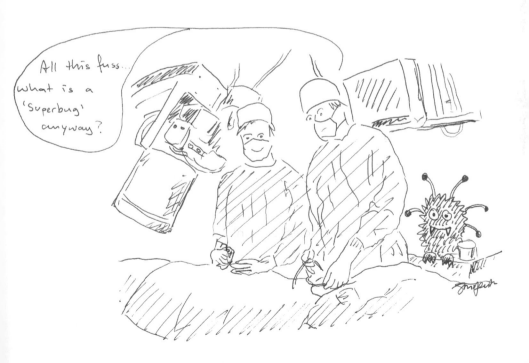

"... is the **idea** that reminding caring **professionals** how to **wash** their **hands** prior to undertaking aseptic procedures, will go some way at least to **slow** the **advance** of this undesirable **organism**."

Now, I've watched the CD, seen the posters and read the pamphlet, so I am now ready to log a 'first' in medical journalism: I am going to wash my mitts right now, prior to stenting this circumflex, and will describe exactly what I do - just as I do it. My words will be recorded verbatim so that you - the reader - will get the sense of being right here with me in the cath lab while I scrub up according to the prescribed protocol. The time you take to read this, will be the same time you should actually take to get scrubbed. OK? Right! Here we go ...

"Our taps are great. You just wave your hand over this sensor and - hold on! Where's my lead coat? [Pause].

"OK, all set! They turn on with a bit of a torrent which can splash up onto your waist. Luckily the lead coat stops it soaking the crutch of my blues, which can take a bit of explaining away otherwise.

"First off - as you will see - no rings, copper bracelets, prayer beads or ancient Egyptian amulets. Hang on! Can you take my watch off? [Pause]. Thanks. Don't put it on that; stick it next to the CD player. And get some music on while you're there.

"So, I rinse both lower arms under the tap letting the water run from my finger tips down to my elbows. Now, after the drips have finished I position the palm of one hand under the nozzle of the antiseptic-soapy

stuff and, with the other forearm, gently depress the plunger of the dispenser while - Bloody Hell! [A dried up piece of crud, crusted around the tip of the spout, has just redirected the jet straight into my left eye. Pause].

"Just keep dabbing it with that swab. Christ, that stings! And wipe the end of that bloody thing as well, will you? Thanks. [Pause].

"OK, I'll need to wet my hands again. [Pause]. There! So, a good helping of this pink stuff and off we go. Initially a circular motion, palm against palm, and then I turn one hand over to do the back ... then the other one. Could someone just scratch the end my nose, please? Up a bit ... lovely! [Pause].

"Now, both wrists and lower arms in turn, making sure we cover the full circumference, then back to the hands so that we can attend to our interdigital clefts. (In microbiological terms, these are the unlit alleyways, the dingy underpasses or the dark passages under railway bridges, where germs hang out; i.e. the spaces between your fingers).

"As you will see (or with any luck at least, imagine), I am not wearing a mask or hat. Observe the way I do each finger individually and then interlock my fingers to ensure that all surfaces are washed. I don't use a nail brush but just for this demonstration, I will. These also come in handy dispensers ... I don't usually do this ... where do I press? Wooops! I'll get another one. Whoa! OK, just leave them there! [Pause].

"Notice that I am keeping splashing to an absolute minimum; a wet cath lab floor is an unsafe - God! Is she alright? [Pause]. Are you OK? Sure? Get the registrar to look at it anyway.

"Rinsing is very important. You need to ensure that the clean water runs downwards from fingertips to elbows. Our taps turn off automatically when they think you have washed for long enough. (For some reason this one is still going, but never mind). When my elbows

have stopped dripping I can turn away from the sink and - Blast! That's dripped right into my clogs.

"Anyway, I carefully take the sterile towel from the gown pack which Staff Nurse has kindly opened for me, and pad up and down until fingers, hands and forearms are dry. I can usually lob this damp, screwed up paper towel straight into that bin from here. Watch this ... so, the Harlem Globetrotters' Meadowlark Lemon goes for the slam dunk ... Oooops! Sorry! Just take it off the trolley, it's sterile.

"On with the gown ... not too tight, thank you ... and lastly the gloves. Different techniques for this, but what you're supposed to do is ... to wiggle your fingers out of the end of the sleeves, and ... ease the glove over your hand and ... Oooh! [Pause].

"Seven-and-a-half please. Can you open them? Just let them drop there. No, there! I've got them. No! I've got them. Not too close! Don't touch me! Damn! [Pause].

"Our taps are great ..."

Chapter 26

The cardiological detective

Dr. Arthur Conan Doyle's famous (fictional?) detective was based on a Professor in his own medical school. Whether we recognise it or not, the practice of medicine incorporates similar investigative skills as we interpret the patient's history, physical signs and test results, in order to reach a conclusion. As a member of the Sherlock Holmes Society of London I therefore submit the following singular narrative. Set in a modern cardiological context, it is a tribute to the 'master' who excelled in the science of deductive reasoning.

The winter of '98 was a memorable one. The city's shivering populous scurried cautiously along slippery pavements and a succession of dawns was greeted with the unmistakable sound of ice being scraped from numerous car windscreens. As a general physician I was pleased to be sitting in clinic with my senior cardiological colleague as we awaited our last client of the morning. Littered with cases of non-cardiac chest pain, palpitation and apparently 'unexplained' breathlessness in impressively obese individuals, it had thus far been a far from stimulating session. I wiped the condensation from the inside of the window and gazed out onto the car park.

"Ah! If I'm not mistaken this looks like our final patient", I mused.

> "... the practice of medicine incorporates similar investigative skills as we interpret the patient's history, physical signs and test results, in order to reach a conclusion."

Holmes peered out into the grey morning and then slumped back into his chair. He placed his slim fingertips together, eased his head back and closed his eyes. "And what do you make of him, Watson?", he sighed, no doubt wishing to test my own observational skills.

"Well", I eagerly responded, "His stick would suggest a likely arthritic condition and his rapid respirations indicate that dyspnoea is likely to be the reason for his attendance."

"Excellent, Watson! Your powers of observation are becoming honed. My cursory glance produced little more data than yours. He is clearly married, an ex-serviceman and a freemason. He lives in the country, has a small dog - probably a terrier - and is a fanatical supporter of Wolverhampton Wanderers. Other than that, I would await closer inspection before theorising further."

"Holmes!" I exploded. "How could you possibly ...?"

"Watson", he soothed, "You see but you do not observe. His wedding ring, British Legion badge and the set square and compasses attached to his watch chain, are obvious enough. Mud on his shoes must mean the country, and teeth marks on the lower end of his stick indicate a dog. Their height from the ground and the hairs on his trouser leg suggest the size and breed. Finally, only a very keen Wolves supporter would go so far as to wear that ludicrously embossed baseball cap.

"As for the referral, you are entirely correct. This hastily scribbled letter from his GP - who is left handed by the way and, judging by this dark brown stain, drinks Lavazza Qualita Rossa espresso coffee - mentions increasing exertional dyspnoea, chest discomfort and the presence of a cardiac murmur."

Our patient entered, tossed his car keys and mobile phone onto the desk and fell gasping into the waiting chair alongside. Within a few minutes Holmes had gleaned the salient features of the history which contributed little more to the information contained in the referral letter.

"You walk your dog less than previously and have gained some weight as a result", he added with a final flourish.

"Exactly, Dr. Holmes, but how could you know?" enquired our patient.

"Elementary!" was the assured response. "You are clearly a keen walker as your shoes, which are undoubtedly of modern fashion, are well worn. However, the symptoms you describe must restrict your activities, and the new hole that you have had to put into your leather belt would indicate that your waist circumference is not as it once was. Now, perhaps you might remove your shirt and vest?"

Watching Holmes examine the patient was spellbinding. His steely blue eyes darted from top to bottom and side to side, scanning the patient's bared torso. His pale hands and quivering spidery fingers moved rapidly over the subject's wrist, neck and praecordium. His stethoscope seemed to appear from nowhere and glide effortlessly over the chest. Each movement would be followed by a few seconds of deep concentration etched onto the chiselled features of the specialist's face.

"Well, Dr. Holmes?", enquired our friend anxiously, as the cardiologist stood erect and sighed with satisfaction.

"You have been to Lanzarote recently, I perceive", Holmes began. The patient blinked with astonishment. "I note that you have been married to your wife, Janet, for 36 years and that you have recently run out of milk. I would also advise that you desist from cigar smoking - King Edwards, if I am not mistaken." The man gasped, but Holmes' calm explanation, as always, engendered reassurance.

"Your sun tan is new and the brightly coloured words on the fob of your car key ring indicate the geographical origin of what I imagine was a souvenir. The adhesive remnants of the price label are still visible indicating that it was purchased recently. The tattoo on your forearm reads Albert and Janet, 1962, and I presume that this is the same 'J' who ends the text message on your mobile phone requesting you not to forget to pick up milk on your way home. As for the cigars, the dusting of ash on your jacket is distinctive, as my monograph on the subject testifies."

"Fantastic!", exclaimed the patient gleefully. "Your reputation as a most skilled consulting cardiologist is entirely justified. But what of my symptoms; have you reached a diagnosis?"

"I have", replied Holmes with a hint of satisfaction. "There is a severe narrowing of your aortic valve and heart surgery is required to replace the valve and rectify the problem." He glanced at me, taking my presence into account as he continued, with a detectable air of boredom. "The murmur is characteristic. The slow rising carotid pulse, sustained and double apical impulse, and the single, soft, second heart sound, leave no room for doubt." He tossed the patient's ECG recording onto the table in front of me and yawned. "The increase in left ventricular voltage and lateral repolarisation changes are simply the icing on the cake."

He turned again to our patient. "I shall arrange echocardiography and cardiac catheterisation for you. You should not have to wait long for these tests on the Health Service. I will also write to your GP. Good morning."

Holmes stood up, thus immediately signifying to the gentleman that the consultation was at an end. The patient was hustled out by our efficient nurse and after the door was shut behind him, Holmes flopped back into his chair. "Well, Watson? Did your own miraculous powers of observation discern anything else that I may have missed?" I could not fail to detect the slightest hint of sarcasm.

"Well ... actually, Holmes", I tentatively began. "There was one thing I noticed that appeared to be of potential importance."

Holmes looked up suddenly, leaned forwards and fixed me with an icy, if not resentful, glare. "Really! And, pray, what might that significant piece of evidence have been?"

"Well, I noticed the top of a letter in his jacket pocket. The light blue capital letters and accompanying ECG logo are distinctive of BUPA, are they not? I deduced that he carries private medical insurance."

Holmes smiled and relaxed back again. His pale cheeks were suddenly tinged with the faintest red and I sensed that beneath his exacting, cold-steel exterior, there dwelt genuine warmth that had been momentarily exposed. My heart swelled with pride; at last I had impressed the master himself.

"Aaah, good old Watson! You are indeed a most loyal and trusted colleague. Be so good as to call our friend back in again for a moment."

Chapter 27

The ties that bind us

It is unavoidable that the following piece will court danger by being seen as a 'man thing'. Nevertheless, I feel obliged to proceed in the interests of healthcare generally and infection control in particular.

A gradually emerging phenomenon concerning male neck wear has been evident for a few years. (Its subtlety may have escaped the larger proportion of gentlemen who leave for work only after the morning ritual of facing a mirror and securing a selected length of material around their neck. The knot - of variable size and shape - is centred directly under their Adam's apple before their shirt collar is turned back down with a triumphant 'flup'. Job done! - dressing was then complete).

Well, not anymore. The days of the neck tie - at least in hospital practice - are numbered.

Its origin, at least in terms of male tailoring fashion, is obscure. I speculate that, perhaps like the waistcoat, it was a device employed by the portly (or 'stout' as defined by M&S) to give a more attractive impression of slimness. The roving eye of the interested female or less interested (hopefully) rival professional male, would begin at the face and then be drawn all too rapidly down the midline under the chin to the lower limbs. Shirt buttons, straining to burst free were hidden from view, and sufficient attention would not be paid to the all too protuberant waist. This ploy would be even more effective if the tie was broad and particularly if flared at its end.

More recently, fashion trends have disguised the original sartorial purpose; whilst the knot might be symmetrical and discretely cover the top shirt button, this arrangement does not apply to TV football pundits or rugby players interviewed fresh from the post match shower. Here the geometry of the knot is more of an irregular rhomboid than a triangle, and the dimensions are sufficient to completely obscure the entire neck (if indeed one was present in the first place).

As for design, there is no limit. We buy, or choose to wear, a particular pattern or motif depending on our mood at the time, but this moment may not necessarily extend into the working day. It is a tad inappropriate, if not a little disconcerting, to have a major set-to about the clinical risk of closing HDU beds with a boardroom full of senior managers, while they can all see the words, "Smile if you're horny", hanging in front of your shirt.

Could it have been Sir Richard-of-Branson, the annoyingly successful entrepreneur, balloonist and modern day 'adventurer', who first prompted this trend? Here is an infinitely wealthy individual, whose slight lack of charisma is made up for by an uncanny resemblance to the classical depiction of Robin Hood, and who chooses to be seen in all aspects of the media, in an open necked shirt and a woolly-pulley. I suspect that robbing the poor to pay the rich allows indulgence in style, although admittedly if he were to sport a patterned silk Hermes and a Windsor knot under his beard, he would indeed look ridiculous.

At meetings more recently, well respected colleagues have appeared - and even indeed, presented - at meetings with the top button of their shirt unfastened. (What the ...?!). You may have also observed that the more flamboyant amongst them have adopted the combination of a jacket over either a polo shirt (acceptable) or, in some cases, a black (usually) T-shirt. The latter combination can look unfortunate as, with the imaginative addition of two cleverly positioned bolts, the result is something akin to Herman Munster.

Dressing etiquette apart, the wearing of ties is now a hot medical topic. Currently hospital managers are seeing ties, in addition to other haute couture, as clothing which may be cleaned sufficiently

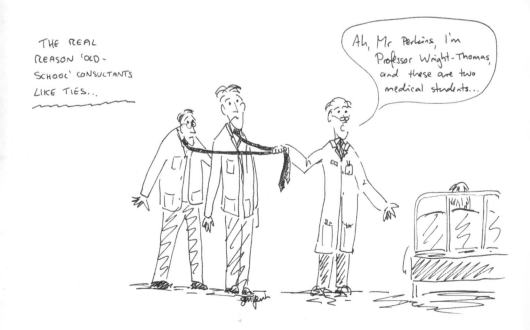

infrequently to potentially provide an infective route of transmission for the more fashion conscious super bug. That is not to deny the practical aspects of such accessories which can disadvantage certain medical specialties; gynaecology and gastroenterology are two well recognised examples in which far sighted (or more likely, short sighted) enthusiasts have taken to sporting bow ties instead.

How is this to impact on cardiology? (Certainly ties have been banned from our cath lab for some time as they often clash with the blue scrubs and get entangled during catheter exchanges). As for the ward, however, I suspect that in the near future we shall see more hygiene-motivated changes, which will not only be confined to our dress sense. White coats, never as crisp, cleansed and starched regularly as originally intended, are a thing of the past. The days of green Medicuts (I guess Venflons are the modern equivalent) gathering dust - and goodness only knows what else - in the top pockets of the 'crash team' are long gone. Perhaps stethoscopes, pens and those old fashioned 'ECG rulers' (remember them?) should be individualised to patients' beds rather than to their attending medics or nurses.

"... hospital managers are seeing ties, in addition to other haute couture, as clothing which may be cleaned sufficiently infrequently to potentially provide an infective route of transmission for the more fashion conscious super bug."

Why stop at neck wear? Suits also may not be dry cleaned as frequently as our infection control matrons may demand. This will require ward-based staff to don scrubs, which is often the case now anyway. Rather than interpret these initiatives as threatening our individual right to express ourselves in the style of our choice, we might instead see such directives as an opportunity to create a whole new NHS clothing range of 'high performance' ward attire. How about snazzy, Trust supplied, polo shirts - sporting an appropriate logo, of course? As with the track suits of football managers, they could also display the wearers' initials, like JM for José Mourinho (just in case a Chelsea striker did not actually know it was his manager yelling at him). On the back and in even larger print, could be embossed words like 'CONS', 'SPR', 'SIS' or 'SOCWR' (social worker, of course), in order to avoid confusion during any frenzied clinical activity on the ward.

So as I write this on New Year's Eve, what might one predict for the 'new man' of 2007? I suspect more undone shirt buttons, an increase in open neck shirts and far fewer ties. Just as long as they are not replaced by medallions.

Chapter 28

A cardiological time capsule

The year is 2107.

Cyborg X300-16R is responsible for the clearing of a derelict Cardiothoracic Centre with a view to thermite demolition and construction of a brand new casino/apartment/prison complex. As the nuclear powered JCB begins to scrape away at the building's foundations, a glint of sunlight is suddenly reflected off an object uncovered for a split second by the huge mechanical claw. It registers as a UVI (Unknown Visual Input) and is relayed back to control. The instruction: "Investigate inappropriate internment" lights up on the cyborg's LED display, positioned where a more anthropomorphic robot designer might have placed the eye sockets instead. Titanium reinforced fingers close around the unearthed box and lift it from the mud, whilst its exterior and contents undergo rapid molecular scanning.

The LED springs into life again, instantaneously transmitting information onto a desk top screen one hundred miles away and viewed by the only human being supervising the rebuilding project: "ID confirmed. Biscuit tin, early 21st century, McVities. Typewritten legend taped on lid. Old English, Times New Roman, twelve point font size. Message reads:

"This box was buried in 2007 AD and contains items or technologies relevant to contemporary cardiological practice. Just as we look back with interest - if not astonishment - and muse at our ancestors' use of burr holes, bleeding and leeches, we can only speculate as to what you will make of the enclosed. Each is accompanied by a personal description."

The human scratches his head and after a short pause sends back instructions to the waiting cyborg: "Continue investigation of contents." Miles away, an extended metal finger cuts a perfect nine inch circle in the tin lid. The resulting superfluous steel disc is vaporised and the mechanical hand then reaches inside to carefully withdraw each item in turn for inspection, photographic documentation and transmission back to base.

Stethoscope

Traditional cardiological device, vital for external detection of otherwise inaudible events occurring during the cardiac cycle and thereby enabling diagnosis to be made at the bedside. More often used simply to identify the holder as a medically qualified individual. Advent of widespread cardiac ultrasound meant that its only residual use was to be able to listen to the patient talking during echocardiography.

ECG recording

Archaic technique that recorded myocardial electrical currents which were detected by electrodes specifically positioned on the chest surface. Certain waveforms became associated with various cardiac pathologies and thereby, together with clinical assessment, directed management strategies, e.g. ST segment elevation: open occluded artery; wiggly line: defibrillate; ST segment depression: sit back and make tea; straight line: call relatives and make tea.

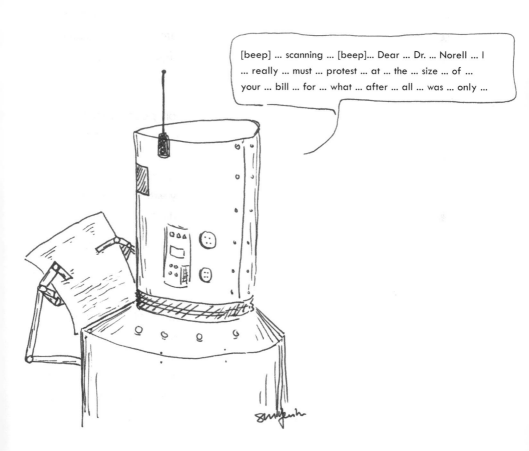

[beep] ... scanning ... [beep]... Dear ... Dr. ... Norell ... I ... really ... must ... protest ... at ... the ... size ... of ... your ... bill ... for ... what ... after ... all ... was ... only ...

Echocardiogram

Non-invasive, painless and entirely safe imaging modality that provided huge amounts of both anatomical and functional information. Because of these qualities it supplanted the resting ECG as the baseline cardiac investigation but unfortunately, in terms of technician time, was far more labour intensive. No matter how much software packages were upgraded, it always retained a quaint degree of subjectivity. In producing reports, check systems were therefore required to ensure that they were clinically relevant. The infamous 'plague of trivial AR' in the early 21st century was the result of such a systems failure.

"Just as we look back with interest - if not astonishment - and muse at our ancestors' use of burr holes, bleeding and leeches, we can only speculate as to what you will make of the enclosed."

Pharmaceuticals (various)

Neuro-endocrine mechanisms, so important in maintaining circulation when we evolved to become land dwelling animals, were found to be deleterious when heart disease prevailed. Hence they were inhibited by beta- and angiotensin-receptor blockers, or converting enzyme inhibitors. We eventually twigged that the platelet was the real villain in acute vascular syndromes, so nearly all the population then took aspirin. Having been born with a cholesterol level at around 1.0, a life time's intake of Macdonalds rapidly jacked this up to 6 or more, resulting in the universal requirement for statins.